A *NEW YORK TIMES* BESTSELLER

"Almond is a shifty cornerback of a writer: rangy, sarcastic, offbeat. And every once in a while, he'll blindside you with a big hit." —DWIGHT GARNER, *THE NEW YORK TIMES*

"An unapologetic, frontal assault on the game's role in American culture." —*LOS ANGELES TIMES*

"[Almond] is a very good writer, and his analysis of problems confronting the game today is well done." —*THE WASHINGTON POST*

"Steve Almond's blistering book *Against Football: One Fan's Reluctant Manifesto* is exactly what it advertises itself to be: an exasperated, frustrated, wide-ranging argument that the time has come to abandon football—particularly but not exclusively the NFL—as a sport built on violence, racism, economic exploitation of poor kids, corrupt dealmaking with local governments over stadiums, and a willingness to find it entertaining to watch people suffer brain damage." —LINDA HOLMES, NPR

"A devastating multi-pronged attack." —*NEWSWEEK*

"Powerful . . . Almond is a sympathetic narrator, his evidence incontrovertible, the moral authority firmly on his side." —*HARPER'S MAGAZINE*

"[Almond's] persuasive book dares fans to consider how long they can continue to ignore football's obvious flaws in order to preserve their weekend ritual." —*BARRON'S*

"*Against Football* is a passionate rant, a devastating case, an ethical plea for sanity, or at least perspective. It's also vintage Steve Almond, fueled by his astonishing wit, intelligence, and decency."
—JESS WALTER, AUTHOR OF *BEAUTIFUL RUINS*

"A passionate and elegantly written book that finally overpowered any rationalization I could come up with to justify watching more football."
—*THE NEW YORK TIMES,*
DEALBOOK

"Almond's book is slim but potent . . . Almond makes his case in a style that is conversational, self-deprecating, sharp and often laugh-out-loud funny."
—*THE PLAIN DEALER*
(CLEVELAND)

"Almond makes it impossible for us to ignore our willing participation in this corrupt and destructive pastime . . . *Against Football* is one fan's inflammatory, yet indispensable, voice in the current conversation about the state of football in America."
—*THE BROOKLYN RAIL*

"*Against Football* . . . makes a strong case that football, as presently practiced by the NFL and NCAA, should be reformed or abolished."
—*THE OREGONIAN* (PORTLAND)

"Almond doesn't pretend to have all the answers, but sometimes it's enough to raise the right questions at the right time. *Against Football* does that with disarming humor and humanity."
—*THE NATIONAL MEMO*

"A book that's part journalism, part memoir, part cultural har-
pooning." —*THE KANSAS CITY STAR*

"There are no easy answers found in Almond's book—and it's an
intentionally provocative argument being made, obviously—but
what it surely does is get you to think about what you're doing
on Sundays, what you're paying to watch and how we could pos-
sibly let children play the game." —*LAS VEGAS WEEKLY*

"A helpful and thoughtful read that traces the criticisms of the
game and the men who run it." —*BITCH MAGAZINE*

"Starting to wonder if it's wrong to watch America's most popu-
lar sport? If children should be allowed to play? You need to read
Against Football by Steve Almond. It's an important book on a
topic that can only get bigger." —GREG EASTERBROOK,
AUTHOR OF *THE KING OF SPORTS:
FOOTBALL'S IMPACT ON AMERICA*

"Pitch-perfect . . . *Against Football* is, at bottom, a love letter from
a heartbroken fan, notable for his eloquence and clarity. It's easy
to imagine that this pungent critique, with quotable passages
on nearly every page, could be a much-needed game-changer. If
that's overly optimistic, then we'll have to settle for a first-rate
piece of journalism and a great read."
—*PORTLAND PRESS HERALD*

"*Against Football* is a book that kicks and prods and fights with
itself and ourselves. Almond is asking himself and us to drop the

ironic distance, open our eyes, and truly look at the dangerous, vile, beautiful, fun, highly corrupted, and horrifically corrupting corporate behemoth we spend so much of our money and leisure time enraptured by, and know what it is that we are doing, and what we are supporting." —*THE MILLIONS*

"Brilliantly states the case for radical change to save the sport." —*TIMES-UNION* (ALBANY)

"Steve Almond's slim but muscular broadside slams into the wall of sanctimonious hokum served up by the NCAA, NFL, and their sycophantic sportswriter enablers." —*POPMATTERS*

"Funny, pained, profane and sharp as a November Saturday in Ann Arbor." —*TAMPA BAY TIMES*

AGAINST FOOTBALL

AGAINST FOOTBALL

ONE FAN'S RELUCTANT MANIFESTO

STEVE ALMOND

WITH A NEW AFTERWORD
BY THE AUTHOR

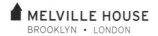

MELVILLE HOUSE
BROOKLYN • LONDON

AGAINST FOOTBALL

Portions of this book originally appeared,
in slightly altered form, in *The New York Times Magazine*.

Melville House Publishing   8 Blackstock Mews
          46 John Street   and   Islington
       Brooklyn, NY 11201   London N4 2BT

mhpbooks.com   facebook.com/mhpbooks   @melvillehouse

ISBN: 978-1-61219-491-2

Library of Congress Control Number: 2014945088

Design by Christopher King

Printed in the United States of America
1 3 5 7 9 10 8 6 4 2

For Peter O. Almond, uncle and hero

"It's a rough business. Because you like watching the game."

—Judah Almond, age five

CONTENTS

PREFACE

I Wasn't Out Cold, But I Was Out   **3**

1. A Brief and Wildly Subjective
   History of Football   **9**
2. A Deep and True Joy Penetrated
   My Being   **24**
3. You Knock My Brains Out This
   Sunday and I Knock Your Brains
   Out the Next Time We Meet   **34**
4. This Eager Violence of the Heart   **58**
5. "Get Money!" on Three   **69**
6. The Love Song of Richie Incognito   **87**
7. The Blind Spot   **104**
8. Their Sons Grow Suicidally Beautiful   **116**
9. All Games Aspire to a Condition
   of War   **133**
10. Bill Simmons Draws the Line   **156**

EPILOGUE

Stop Being a Fan, Start Being a Player   **173**

Sudden Death: An Odd but
Necessary Afterword   **179**

Acknowledgments   **193**

AGAINST FOOTBALL

I WASN'T OUT COLD, BUT I WAS OUT

Among the motley artifacts taped to the walls of my office—tucked below the photo of the Bay City Rollers in snug tartan jumpsuits and the student evaluation that reads, "If writing were a part of my body, I would cut it off with an Exacto blade"—is a tiny yellowed clipping.

It's a grand total of two paragraphs, snipped from a *Boston Globe* recap of the New England Patriots' 12–0 win over the Miami Dolphins on December 7, 2003. I'm almost certain I didn't watch this contest, because I hate the Patriots, though oddly, if I'm honest (which I don't like being in the context of my sports-viewing habits) I have watched *a lot* of Pats games over the years, so there's a decent chance I caught a portion of this one, maybe just the third quarter at a friend's house.

The passage reads:

> *With 13 minutes 50 seconds left in the game, running back Kevin Faulk hauled in a 15-yard pass from quarterback Tom Brady, then got leveled by Miami safety Brock Marion, who forced a fumble and left Faulk motionless on the ground.*
>
> *"I wasn't out cold, but I was out," said Faulk. Asked if*

he remembered lying on the ground, he said, "No, I don't, so I must have been out. I knew that something was wrong with me. I knew that, like, it wasn't normal. I didn't have that same, normal feeling when I got up."

I have no idea how I came across this dispatch. I don't subscribe to the *Globe*, so I probably found it on the subway. I do remember the strange buzz that accompanied the reading of these words. The first paragraph is standard sports reportage: game data, a stark description of collision and injury. But that second paragraph! It read more like a poignant existential monologue. Faulk seeks to minimize his injury, then, pressed, struggles to assimilate what happened to him, which most physicians would describe as a significant injury to the brain. What you're hearing is the linguistic equivalent of a concussion.

I thought it was funny.

That would be the simplest way to explain why I brought this story home and cut out the section in question and taped it to my wall. I thought it said something elemental about athletic delusion, the absurd and pitiful way players hide from the truth of their vocation: that they earn ungodly sums of money and acclaim for demolishing each other.

I assumed, in other words, a posture of ironic distance, which is what we Americans do to avoid the corruption of our spiritual arrangements. Ironic distance allows us to separate ourselves from the big, complicated moral systems around us (political, religious, familial), to sit in judgment of others rather than ourselves. It's the reason, as we zoom into the twilight years of our imperial reign, that Reality TV has become our designated guilty pleasure.

But here's the thing: You can run from your own subtext for only so long. Those spray-tanned lunatics we happily revile are merely turned-out versions of our private selves, the whores we hide from public view.

What I mean is that there's a deeper reason I cut those paragraphs out of the paper a dozen years ago, and carried that little square of newsprint with me through three different moves, each time affixing it to a spot right over my desk.

I told myself it was just a macabre little talisman, a window into the dissonant psyches of famous barbarians. Then, a few months ago, around the time my own mother suffered an acute and terrifying insult to her brain, the truth landed. The passage wasn't about Faulk and his brethren. It was about me. It was about the forty years I'd spent as an ardent football fan, about my refusal to face the complicity of my own joy in seeing men like Kevin Faulk concussed.

I knew that something was wrong with me.

The game in which Faulk got hurt took place in the midst of an historic fifteen-game win streak that would carry the

Patriots to their second Super Bowl in three seasons. The moment captured was, by the standards of gridiron lore, the zenith of that team's fortunes. The only extant photo of the play shows Marion colliding with Faulk in helmet-to-helmet fashion. Both men are grimacing. Marion's knee appears to be striking the helmet of a third figure, Miami linebacker Junior Seau, who is grasping at Faulk from the ground.

In 2012, nine years after this play and two years into retirement, Seau would fire a .357 Magnum into his chest. Although never diagnosed with a concussion during his twenty-year career, an autopsy of his brain would reveal chronic brain damage.

This little book is a manifesto. Its job is to be full of obnoxious opinions. For example, I happen to believe that our allegiance to football legitimizes and even fosters within us a tolerance for violence, greed, racism, and homophobia.

I recognize that voicing these opinions will cause many fans to write off whatever else I might have to say on the subject as a load of horseshit, shoveled by someone who is probably wearing a French sailor's suit and whistling the Soviet National Anthem.

Before you do so, let me reiterate: I am one of you. If we ever have the awkward pleasure of meeting, we can, rather than debating my obnoxious opinions about football, happily muse over any of the hundreds of NFL players, past and present, whose names and career paths and highlight reels I have, pathetically, unintentionally, and yet lovingly, filed away in my hippocampal hard drive. Chances are I know all about your favorite team, what they did last year and last decade and whom they drafted (at least in the first round) and where they're predicted to finish in their division, a subject I would prefer to take up, given the alternative, which would be to discuss my team, the wretched and moribund Oakland Raiders, who will finish this season—mark my words—no better than 3–13.

So please, before you set this book down, or quietly remit it to the poor soul in your life who thought it might make an "interesting" gift, please consider one final obnoxious opinion: I happen to believe that football, in its exalted moments, is not just a sport but a lovely and intricate form of art.

Mostly, this book is a personal attempt to connect the two disparate synapses that fire in my brain when I hear the word "football": the one that calls out, *Who's playing? What channel?*, and the one that murmurs, *Shame on you.* My hope is to honor the ethical complexities *and* the allure of the game. I'm trying to see football for what it truly is.

What does it mean that the most popular and unifying form of entertainment in America circa 2014 features giant muscled men, mostly African-American, engaged in a sport that causes many of them to suffer brain damage? What does it mean that our society has transmuted the intuitive physical joys of childhood—run, leap, throw, tackle—into a corporatized form of simulated combat? That a collision sport has become the leading signifier of our institutions of higher learning, and the undisputed champ of our colossal Athletic Industrial Complex?

I knew that, like, it wasn't normal.
So what was it?

Steve Almond
Arlington, Massachusetts
April 2014

1

A BRIEF AND WILDLY SUBJECTIVE HISTORY OF FOOTBALL

I believe in ... rough, manly sports. I do not feel any particular sympathy for the person who gets battered about a good deal so long as it is not fatal.

—President Theodore Roosevelt

Football began, more or less, as a series of controlled riots. The earliest variations were staged in the 1820s at elite Eastern colleges, often as a class rush designed to visit harm upon incoming freshman. "Boys and young men knocked each other down," the *New York Evening Post* observed. "Eyes were bunged, faces blacked and bloody, and shorts and coats torn to rags." The brawls grew so destructive that both Yale and Harvard banned the game in 1860.

But restless student athletes continued to assemble teams, eventually challenging other schools to contests that combined elements of soccer and rugby. Representatives met to establish common rules. The line of scrimmage replaced the scrum, a crucial adjustment that granted one team uncontested possession of the ball. A set of downs followed, then a scoring system.

The game remained astonishingly brutal. The only way to advance the ball was for players to lock arms and smash their bare heads against an equally determined and unprotected opposition. In 1904, eighteen players died, most of them prep school boys. Scores more suffered gruesome injuries: wrenched spinal cords, fractured skulls, broken ribs. Editorialists decried football as an abomination unworthy of civil society.

When word reached Theodore Roosevelt in the Oval Office that his alma mater, Harvard, was again considering outlawing the game, he vowed to "minimize the danger," though not so much that the game would be played "on too ladylike a basis." Roosevelt, whose own son had his nose broken playing for Harvard, convened a summit of football authorities. Reforms followed forthwith.

The mass formations, essentially human battering rams, were prohibited. A neutral zone between offense and defense was established, along with a more sophisticated mechanism to advance the ball: a team had to gain 10 yards in three downs. The most radical change was the legalization of the forward pass. A game heretofore restricted to one thudding plane was suddenly, miraculously, bestowed a z-axis. The ball could be sent spiraling over a helpless opponent. In 1913, Norte Dame used its superior passing game to upset a heavily favored and much larger Army team, a contest regarded as the birth of the modern game.

In a spatial sense, football shifted from a mass of heaving bodies to an ornate and calibrated set of formations—double wing, split-T, wishbone, shotgun—that required a division of labor. A clear hierarchy emerged. The quarterback led the offense. He called the plays, took the snap, then handed off to bruising running backs or threw to wiry flankers, while hulking linemen cloistered him from assault. Defenses countered by diversifying into nose tackles, linebackers, safeties.

Speed, agility, and subterfuge took their places alongside brute strength as the game's abiding virtues. For teams to be successful, players had to move in concert, which meant practice, coordination, a growing sense of interdependence. They had to react to multiple contingencies on each play. These strategic demands soon required the introduction of a managerial figure, the coach.

Walter Camp, the game's most famous early champion, regarded football as a form of "purposeful work" that evolved from the chaotic play of rugby. It is easy enough to see the parallels to industrialization here. Football may be the most striking example of incremental innovation in American history.

But something more fundamental was going on as well: the creation of beauty and meaning from controlled violence. The anarchy of a folk game had been shaped into an organized sport, carefully refined, made more coherent and complex. The excessive savagery of football's origins became the engine of its transformation and thus its saving grace.

•　•　•

Much has been written about the uniquely American quality of football. It is the only major sport that proceeds as a series of marches into enemy territory. It combines ground and aerial assaults. It is the athletic equivalent of manifest destiny. And so on.

A lot of this stuff is hokum, a kind of overheated historiography meant to boil down the complicated origins and growth of this country, and its diverse population, into a single "American" mindset. But the fact remains: in the space of a century football grew from an obscure collegiate hazing ritual into the nation's most popular professional sport.

Why?

In *Reading Football: How the Popular Press Created an American Spectacle*, his revelatory book about the early years of the game, cultural theorist and former NFL player Michael Oriard offers a set of interlocking theories:

"With industrialization, the closing of the frontier, and the migration to the cities, the American male was cut off from the physical demands of everyday outdoor life," Oriard writes. "Thrust into a new world where traditional masculine traits were no longer meaningful, he found vigorous outdoor sports such as football a compensating validation of his manhood."

Consider the plight of a young man born in Chicago or Pittsburgh or San Francisco at the turn of the century. His parents or grandparents were pioneers. Yet he's trapped in some sooty factory or office or slaughterhouse. Toward what diversion might he turn to feel his physical yearnings expressed, to banish the feeling of urban anonymity?

Oriard argues further that football's rich narrative structure allowed sportswriters to convey the thrill of the game, its suspense and artistry, to a mass audience. One such scribe, Heywood Broun, compared football to the stories of O. Henry. "First come the signals of the quarterback. This is the preliminary exposition," he explained. "Then the plot thickens, action becomes intense and a climax is reached whereby the mood of tragedy or comedy is established."

Fans found in football an irresistible duality. It was at once mythic and visceral, liberating and lethal, Eros and Thanatos rolled into one compact drama.

The size of live crowds swelled. By the 1890s, big games drew up to 40,000 fans. This being America, before long fans of means recognized that there was money to be made. Oriard puts it like this: "Football succeeded as spectacle because the games' own structure made narrative drama possible, but also because these narrative possibilities were exploited by football's promoters."

Football historians have a tendency to cite certain games as watersheds. The 1958 championship, in which the upstart Baltimore Colts, led by Johnny Unitas, beat the New York Giants in overtime, is known as "The Greatest Game Ever Played." Or Broadway Joe Namath steering the New York Jets past the insurmountable Colts a decade later, in Super Bowl III. But a far more pivotal contest took place in 1925, when the Pottsville Maroons, champions of the fledgling

NFL, upset a squad of Notre Dame all-stars and thus established the league's legitimacy against the dominant college game. This was the crucial first step in transforming an extracurricular activity into a popular for-profit enterprise.

People tend to overlook the fact that pro football entered the twentieth century as a heavy underdog to baseball and boxing, which dominated the sporting landscape. The NFL managed to survive these lean years for three key reasons.

First, the owners, many of them former players, were intensely loyal to the game. Second, they were shrewd and (if necessary) pitiless businessmen. Third, and most surprising, they viewed the league as a collective endeavor that would require shared sacrifice, an attitude generally rare amongst men of privilege.

Owners of less prosperous teams routinely lost tens of thousands of dollars each year. Despite these setbacks, most stuck with the league. They understood that the popularity of the college game had created a market for the pros, along with a built-in labor pool that included national stars such as Red Grange. And they accepted that the NFL would survive only if all of its teams remained competitive and solvent. They worked together to outflank and eventually absorb rival startups, and approved a number of egalitarian innovations.

League schedules, for instance, pitted the weak against the weak and the strong against the strong early in the season—a scheme designed to keep teams in contention for as long as possible. Owners would later jigger with the college draft to achieve the same end, allowing the worst clubs to select first.

Finally, the NFL, following the example of its erstwhile rivals in the AFL, eventually decided to structure its television deals so that all teams received an equal share.

To be clear: the owners who agreed to these measures were, as a rule, extraordinarily rich men intent on becoming more so. But they also knew that unleashing the hounds of capitalism would create a pigskin version of the New York Yankees, which would lead to poorer teams going under, which, in turn, would doom the whole endeavor.

Football enjoyed other crucial advantages in the emergent marketplace of American fandom. The pace and the temperament of the game resonated with a rapidly industrializing culture. Baseball, measured against its younger rival, felt meandering, pastoral, restrained.

It was football that managed to pluck at the American tension between violence and self-control, brains and brawn, ferocity and grace, individual stardom and communal achievement, between painstaking preparation and the instant of primal release. The action was simple enough to appeal to a child, the strategy dense enough to engage men of learning.

And, of course, television changed everything.

To say that TV has been good for football would be like saying that roads have been good for cars. Most Americans had never seen a football game until television showed them one. Games were rare, geographically isolated events (particularly in contrast to baseball, with its 162-game season and countless minor leagues).

Television proved the ideal medium for revealing the pleasures of football to a mass audience. Cameras framed and magnified the action. The complex mayhem of the game, the jarring collisions, all became simultaneously more intimate and abstract. Commentators helped make sense of what viewers were seeing. Intense bursts were followed by reflective lulls. Drives lent a dramatic structure to the game. But because a team could lose possession on any given play, there was a fluid quality to the action. Fans were subjected to what behavioral psychologists would recognize as a variable reinforcement schedule. There was always the chance that a play would break big, that a runner would slash into the open field, or that a receiver would nab a pass and head for daylight. Or, best of all, that some unforeseeable calamity—a blocked punt, an interception returned for a touchdown— would swing the momentum.

Football also managed to hit the Goldilocks zone when it came to scoring: there was enough to keep fans engaged, but not so much as to make it seem routine. The winding down of the clock served to ratchet up suspense in close games. There were even timeouts for snacks and bathroom breaks.

Perhaps most important, the sly handiwork of multiple cameramen and skilled editors intensified the visual impact of each contest, bringing into focus intricacies and eliciting emotional valences that might otherwise have been lost. Don DeLillo put it like this: "In slow motion the game's violence became almost tender, a series of lovely and sensual assaults. The camera held on fallen men, on men about to be hit, on those who did the hitting. It was a loving relationship with just a trace of mockery; the camera lingered a bit too long, making poetic sport of the wounded."

By the sixties, pro football had surpassed baseball as the nation's top spectator sport. Not only did it flourish on television, but with the print media as well. "I'm developing a strong hunch that pro football is our sport," noted André Laguerre, the managing editor of *Sports Illustrated*, in 1962. "We have grown with it, and each of us is a phenomenon of the times." Laguerre deemed the college game "too diffuse and regionalized" and baseball "old-fashioned."

Under the guidance of its young, media-savvy commissioner, Pete Rozelle, the league made several prescient decisions. It created a division called NFL Properties, which brought interests such as merchandising and promotions in-house. The league recognized, long before its competition, that America had become an information economy, and it flooded media outlets with stats and player profiles.

Rozelle was essentially a PR man, and he understood the American lust for the mythic, the manner in which his fellow citizens yearned to feel part of some heroic past. In 1965, he convinced the owners to create NFL Films, which amounted to a ministry of propaganda. The highlight reels produced by this outfit were wildly ambitious cinematic productions that featured bloody linemen, frozen breath, and floating spirals, all set to a rousing score, and narrated by a voice actor whose flair for gravitas fell somewhere between Captain Kirk and Darth Vader. It is virtually impossible to watch one of these films without feeling engorged by delirious notions of valor. They are football porn.

Given the game's appeal to traditional masculine values, it's hardly surprising that men of power gravitated to the game, nor that the ad executives of the world understood its lucrative associations. What remains shocking is the vast reach of the game, the manner in which it united low and high culture, the egghead and the meathead, the radical and the reactionary, the proletariat and the President.

Eisenhower played the game, as did Jack and Bobby Kennedy, rather famously. But it was Richard Nixon whose fanaticism was most blatant. In 1969, Nixon telephoned quarterback Len Dawson minutes after he led the Kansas City Chiefs to a startling win in Super Bowl IV. (Informed that he had a call from the President, Dawson responded, "The president of what?") Nixon spiked his campaign speeches with football jargon. He used gridiron nomenclature to nickname military operations. He didn't just go to games. He visited the *practices* of his favorite team, the Washington Redskins.

The scene I can't get out of my head is of Nixon milling around outside the broadcast booth at a 1971 pre-season game, waiting to do a brief televised chat with Frank Gifford, the former Giants star turned broadcaster. Nixon can't stop talking about how he used to watch Gifford play, how he attended the Giff's post-game cocktail parties. This is the most powerful man on earth, still three years from his appointed disgrace, and he is unable to settle his nerves. "I know Frank Gifford," he says. "I'm sure he'll remember me."

The NFL marketed football as a traditional game, shaped by Establishment values. The league was both a friend to big business and a crucial partner. It had survived its precarious infancy largely by adopting the tactics of the emerging corporate culture.

But it wasn't just Nixon and the rest of the squares who loved football. Here's what Abbie Hoffman, the most famous dissident of the sixties, had to say about football haters: "They're a bunch of peacenik creeps. Watching a football game on television, in color, is fantastic." This is to say nothing of the Black Panthers, who gathered on Sunday afternoons to watch at a bar owned by hall of famer Gene Upshaw, or George Plimpton, who devoted two books to the game.

"Football is not only the most popular sport, it is the most intellectual one. It is in fact the intellectuals' secret vice," the critic William Phillips observed in 1969. "Much of its popularity is due to the fact that it makes respectable the most primitive feelings about violence, patriotism, manhood."

A more generous way of saying this is that football provided a lingua franca by which men of vastly different beliefs and standing could speak to one another in an increasingly fragmented culture. It cut right through the moral ambiguities and antagonisms of the era.

Consider the one and only meeting between President Nixon and his counter-cultural bane, Hunter S. Thompson. The two spent most of the hour swapping game stories, after which Thompson noted, with reluctant admiration, "Whatever else might be said about Nixon—and there is still serious doubt in my mind that he could pass for human—he is a goddamn stone fanatic on every facet of pro football."

The British writer James Lawton puts it this way: "If all sport is magnificent triviality, American football seems least tolerant of its limitations."

It is hard to imagine this today, but there was a time when interest in football was restricted to weekend afternoons in the autumn. Today, the amount of time that fans spend watching games is infinitesimal compared to the time we spend consuming what might be called the ancillary products: highlights, previews, updates on injuries, trades, arrests, contract negotiations, firings, and so on. This is to say nothing of the message boards and the endless chatter of sports pundits, the arias of wrath intended to fill the overnight hours of sports talk radio. Americans now give football more attention than any other cultural endeavor. It isn't even close.

The result (in sports, as in any other racket) is an obscene inflationary bubble. An errant comment on Twitter begets a national story and weeks of agitated kibitzing, and a player accused of something more serious—dogfighting or murder—commands the grave regard once reserved for a presidential scandal.

The NFL and the networks that cover the college game have tapped into a bottomless hunger for which there is no off-season. The moment the Super Bowl ends, draft speculation begins. The draft itself wasn't even televised until a few years ago. More than 25 million people watched the first round last year. At Ohio State, where I happen to be teaching as I write this, more than 80,000 people will fill the stadium . . . for a spring scrimmage.

If you are among the thousands of handicappers who make a living from gambling on football, or the millions who place bets, the desire for minute and esoteric bytes of football info strikes me as understandable.

For the rest of us, I suspect, this data mongering has more to do with a dire search for meaning. Let me try to explain. Americans are being bombarded by facts at this point in our history. Sea levels rose 3.2 millimeters last year. The Nikkei average is down 6 percent. Dick Cheney remains sentient. The problem isn't that these facts are bad, though most are. It's that we have no larger context in which to place them. We don't really know what they mean.

The reason I'll spend five minutes reading about whether the second-string running back for the Arizona Cardinals is going to show up for training camp is because that fact plugs into a system of loyalties I do understand. As absurd as this sounds, it *means* something to me. The Raiders play the Cardinals this year . . . if their first-string running back gets injured, perhaps their second-stringer will be ill-prepared . . . meaning our feeble defense might stymie him . . . and so forth.

The glut of football news also feeds a kind of vicarious executive impulse. We live in an age of unfettered capitalism, and yet most of us know next to nothing about the true mechanisms of economic power. We can barely remember the PINs to our 401(k)s. When it comes to football, though, we have access to vast stores of financial and personnel data, scouting reports, statistical analyses, game tapes, the works. There is no way on earth we could run IBM or General Electric, nor would most of us want to. But we could sure as shit do a better job with the Dallas Cowboys than their jackass owner Jerry Jones. This is why so many millions of Americans spend so many billions of hours deliberating over whom to start each week on their fantasy football rosters.

How much bigger can football get? I was thinking about this, inappropriately, a few months ago in church.

I am not a regular churchgoer. But our family attends the local Unitarian Universalist service when we can get our act together, mostly so we can feel a part of some community that still believes in social justice and economic equality and the rest of those extinct hippie values.

Anyway, what happened was that the reverend mentioned football. He told us that the last time he'd delivered this particular sermon, the Patriots had lost their playoff game that afternoon. So it wasn't even a formal part of his talk; it was an ad-lib. And it got by far the biggest response of anything he said. The instant he made this joke, the whole congregation, maybe a hundred of us, laughed and nodded. We had something in common.

Naturally, I started thinking about the game he had mentioned, which I had watched with bitter glee, and began recapping it in my head. Then I looked around and thought: *Wow. Even in the UU.* Then I thought about John Lennon and how he said the Beatles were bigger than Jesus and how much grief he got for telling that particular truth. Then I thought about how many people were going to watch the Patriots game that afternoon, or some other football game, and how that number might compare to the number of people who attended a church or a synagogue or a mosque. What would that ratio be? Five to one?

Then I thought about the amount of time Americans, men in particular but also women, spend thinking about football during a given week, as opposed to thinking about God and the state of our souls and whether we are leading a noble life, and I realized that I probably spent about ten minutes max on these issues, whereas my recap of the Patriots game had already run fifteen or more. I thought about the tens of millions of fans—the tailgaters, the face painters—whose sacred wishes and fears and prayers are reserved for a vicious and earthly game.

Then I thought: *Shit. That's me, isn't it?*

2

A DEEP AND TRUE JOY PENETRATED MY BEING

I'm going to start in a dark place and work my way toward the light.

So: I'm a lifelong Oakland Raiders fan.

Confessing this publicly to anyone who knows anything about the NFL is like revealing that I'm the son of two psychoanalysts, which also happens to be true. I can tell exactly what other people are thinking, whether or not they ever say it out loud. They are thinking: this guy is a fucking nut.

For those who are not familiar with the Raiders, they are the epitome of the term *once proud*, a franchise incapable of accepting that its best years are past. I think of them as the NFL's version of a wildly popular child actor who starred in a couple of minor hits in the eighties and has now grown into an ugly, entitled, coke-addicted adult who struts around D-list parties in mirrored sunglasses and parachute pants reeking of Polo cologne and insulting the women who decline his invitation to head back to his pad to check out his python.

There is some chance I have given this analogy too much thought.

The point is that the Raiders were very good when I was young and that they have been very bad for the past decade, the laughingstock of the NFL, such that they are best known at present not for any actual players but for their most exuberant fans, who smear their faces with silver and black and (for no clear reason) wear tunics with spikes and dog collars and other vaguely post-apocalyptic accouterments.

I started watching them at about age five. We lived in a sleepy suburb an hour south of San Francisco, but the 49ers were terrible. The Raiders were where the action was. They were giant and swaggering. I was small and cowering. The psychic math was not especially hard to do.

Mostly, I wanted to be close to my dad. That's why most boys take up with sports. Teamwork, dedication, killer instinct—all that stuff comes later. In the beginning, you just want to be with your dad. And that's what football got me, every Sunday afternoon. We'd hang a thick wool blanket over the curtain rod in the TV room to cut the glare and watch Kenny "The Snake" Stabler hobble around on his ruined knees and throw his lovely ducks to Cliff Branch and Freddy Biletnikoff. We watched Mark van Eeghen blast into the line maybe a million times, gaining 2 yards the hard way. We watched All-Pro linebacker Ted Hendricks wield his forearm like a truncheon, and cornerback Lester Hayes patrol the secondary so extravagantly festooned with a snot-colored adhesive called Stickum as to appear leprous. We watched a bald, ill-tempered obelisk by the name of Otis Sistrunk descend upon quarterbacks like a slow and final doom.

We watched the Raiders dismantle the Vikings in Super Bowl XI and squeak by the Chargers in the playoffs on a last-second fluke fumble that was batted and punched and kicked into the end zone then fallen upon by the sure-handed tight end Dave Casper.

I was the only hardcore fan in our house, the only one who submitted to the narcotic absurdity of the arrangement, who allowed the wins and losses to become personal. It was how I coped with the competitive angst of having two brothers who were bigger and stronger than me. I handed my fate over to the Raiders. I let them do the dirty work.

Later on, I adapted. I started playing sports myself, well enough to make a few teams. I experimented with mild forms of delinquency and smoked huge amounts of pot and ate my weight in low-grade candy and (Lord help me) used the family hot tub as a masturbatory aide. I took the SATs then I took them again and shipped off to a liberal arts college where being a football fan seemed to connote a tragic lack of imagination.

So I left the game behind for a while.

That's bullshit, of course. I never did any such thing. I was still rooting through the dry soil of the box scores, tracking the Raiders' descent into mediocrity while pretending I had better things to do. These better things included interning in the sports department of my hometown newspaper, and later becoming a sportscaster for the campus radio station.

Somewhere in the world, I'm afraid, there exists a recording of me providing the color commentary for a game in which we bowed to our rivals 56–0, a score that makes the game sound closer than it was.

Then I was in El Paso, working at a newspaper and living with a woman who considered football an unfortunate symptom of patriarchal thought systems. I was trying to take myself more seriously. That's how I wound up in the sarcophagal sub-basement of the El Paso Public Library, where they stashed the fiction and where, one day, I came across a novel by Don DeLillo called *End Zone*, which I picked up for the simple reason that the front cover featured a football.

It came as a pleasant shock that the book was actually *about* football, and more so that it was set in West Texas. This seemed like a very big deal to me. It encouraged the delusion—always so tantalizing to the chronically self-involved—that there was some cosmic connection between the text and myself.

End Zone's narrator is Gary Harkness, a running back who winds up at tiny Logos College to evade the draft board and settle his addled brain. "Whatever complexities, whatever dark politics of the human mind, the heart—these are noted only within the chalked borders of the playing field," Harkness assures us. "At times strange visions ripple across the turf; madness leaks out. But wherever else he goes, the football player travels the straightest of lines. His thoughts are wholesomely commonplace, his actions uncomplicated by history, enigma, holocaust or dream."

I had no idea what this meant. But I loved *End Zone* for its descriptions of football, passages in which the sensual experience of the game generated a hallucinogenic intensity. "On a spring-action trap I went straight ahead," Harkness says, "careened off 77 and got leveled by Mike Mallon. He came down on top of me, breathing into my face, chugging like a train. I closed my eyes. The noise of the crowd seemed miles away. Through my jersey the turf felt chilly and hard. I heard somebody sigh. A deep and true joy penetrated my being. I opened my eyes. All around me there were people getting off the ground. Directly above were the stars, elucidations in time, old clocks sounding their chimes down the bending universe."

I had never thought about football as a transcendent experience. I'd accepted the allegedly more enlightened view that it was a diversion from the serious business of adulthood, and that my fandom represented a shameful refusal to leave childhood behind. But the exquisite renderings of football in *End Zone* suggested a richer possibility: that sport awakens within us deep recesses of emotion, occasions for reflection, reasons to believe.

Late in the novel, Harkness and his teammates play a pickup game in the driving snow. It quickly degenerates into a free-for-all. "We were adrift within this time and place and what I experienced then, speaking just for myself, was some variety of environmental bliss," he observes. "We were getting extremely basic, moving into elemental realms, seeking harmony with the weather and the earth." This was the novel's thrashing heart: an ecstatic celebration of the body at play.

Passages like this sent me reeling back to my own youth, to the game we played every day at recess and after school. Tackle the Pill had one rule: bring down the kid with the football. You didn't even need a ball. Some days we played with an empty milk carton. And what I loved about the game were the revelations of momentum and leverage, the way an abrupt reversal of direction would send a tackler slingshotting past, and you would burst into the clear, adrenaline fizzing beneath your ribs, the next tackler taking his angle and some ancient instinct within you already working out how to make him miss—stutter step, spin, straight-arm, all three synced and firing in sequence—and always the need to keep those knees churning, especially if someone grabbed your shirt, to churn toward that magical trice when your centrifugal energy ripped his grip loose and sent his body hurtling out of your orbit like a satellite hitting escape velocity.

This was football distilled to its essence: You think you can tackle me. Go ahead. Try.

Emmett Creed, the gnomic coach in *End Zone*, puts it like this:

> *"People stress the violence. That's the smallest part of it. Football is brutal only from a distance. In the middle of*

it there's a calm, a tranquility. The players accept pain. There's a sense of order even at the end of a running play with bodies strewn everywhere. When the systems inter-lock, there's a satisfaction to the game that can't be dupli-cated. There's a harmony."

Creed was right. I loved the pileups, the sensation of be-ing crushed by the weight of my loyal enemies. The rules dictated that some other boy would have to grab the ball and set off. But a few times a game, after a long run, there would be a stillness where by some unspoken assent we could briefly retire from the hard work of being boys, all the fight-ing and feinting, the pretending not to be afraid, where we consented to be joined in these secret burdens, a dozen broth-ers pressed against each other and the earth in an unembar-rassed embrace.

It's true: we accepted the pain. I can remember being knocked cold in a game with some bigger kids and staggering home from Los Robles Park with a knot above my eye and a thumping headache, livid they wouldn't let me keep play-ing. I was probably nine. At a sleepover in seventh grade, we snuck out for a midnight game and Steve Hayes tripped on a sprinkler head and broke his arm and we got his best friend to walk him home so his dad could drive him to the emergency room so we could finish the contest.

During a pickup game in high school, in a drenching rain, someone came up under my arm and lurched me out of bounds. I walked back to the huddle with a peculiar sensation of tightness on the right side of my upper torso then heard a dull *pop*, which was the ball of my shoulder joint slipping back into its socket. The same thing happened again a few plays later. It never occurred to me to stop playing.

Much of this was the invincible idiot joy of youth. But there's something about football that elicits this behavior. You know you might get hurt playing. That's part of *why* you play, to see what you're made of, how you take a hit, to see what happens when your courage meets real hazard.

In high school, I began showing up outside Stanford Stadium on Saturday mornings so I could sell hot dogs at the football games. This involved lugging around a giant steel box heated by two cans of Sterno and filled with hot dogs wrapped in white paper, a set-up that led to blistered hands and several small fires.

I loved the job. Stanford wasn't much good in the early eighties, but they had an all-world quarterback named John Elway. He was almost comically handsome, a blond, horse-jawed kid who ambled around with a pigeon-toed grace. If Johnny Unitas were crossbred with Zeus the result would be John Elway. He threw so hard in practice his receivers all bore identical bruises on their sternums: a tiny purple x where the seams of the ball met.

The play I've never forgotten from that era was a third-and-long from midfield. Elway's offensive line broke down, as it did most plays, and he rolled out to his left, where a blitzing linebacker awaited him. He zipped back to his right only to encounter more rushers and reversed field again. At this point, he had retreated some 25 yards and was being chased by a conga-line of homicidal defenders. It was a strange sequence. What happens, I wondered, if the quarterback *never stops going backward*? If he exits the field of play? The stadium? The municipality? What's the penalty in that situation? We never found out. Because Elway did something categorically insane. He wheeled around and cocked his throwing arm, even as his antagonists closed in.

I should note that the mood in the stadium at this point was one of concerted dread. Nothing good was going to happen on this play. Elway had done something very stupid and his punishment was likely to include the cracking of his bones and the sucking of his marrow.

But there is a reason that John Elway was down on that field and we were sitting in the stands. Elway knew the capacities of his body. He knew (or at least believed) that he could throw a football 80 yards in the air off his back foot as he was about to get steamrolled. And the amazing, almost spooky thing, is that one of his receivers knew this too, because he was standing on the opposing team's goal line waiting as Elway let fly. He waited for what seemed to all of us a very long few seconds, as the ball fell out of the sky and into his cradled arms. No defender was anywhere near him. It was like watching an outfielder shag a lazy fly ball.

I remember also that the old Stanford stadium had this little patch of grass off to the side of the end zone where kids could scrimmage. And during the next timeout, I watched a bunch of boys I knew—they were members of my soccer team, actually—attempt to recreate the play, over and over.

That's what kids do. We're a mimetic species. We see greatness and we try to locate a version of it in our own bodies.

We all recognized what John Elway had done on that field. He might have been any kid on any playground. Elway ran around like crazy until he spotted something nobody else did, a path to redemption where others saw only ruin. In the moment of greatest peril, he summoned poise. In the midst of entropy, he found order. We all want to find that magic within ourselves. And failing that, we want to watch as someone else does.

3

YOU KNOCK MY BRAINS OUT THIS SUNDAY AND I KNOCK YOUR BRAINS OUT THE NEXT TIME WE MEET

And if that's all there was to football, well, we could stop right here and go stock up on snacks for this weekend's games. But of course I've left the ugly parts out of this highlight reel. I've failed to mention, for instance, the single most haunting memory of my childhood fandom.

In the summer of 1978, during a pre-season game, a wide receiver for the New England Patriots named Darryl Stingley lunged for a pass just out of his reach. Before he could regain his balance he was leveled by Raiders defensive back Jack Tatum. It was clear at once that Stingley was, in the gentle parlance of the broadcast booth, "shaken up on the play." Team doctors rushed to his side.

I was eleven years old. I knew I was supposed to feel bad for Stingley, and I did in some minor, dutiful way. Mostly I was proud of Tatum, of the destructive capacities central to his identity. The whole point of being Jack "The Assassin" Tatum was to poleax wide receivers in this manner.

The problem was that Stingley wasn't moving. The doctors kept tapping at his knees with reflex hammers and I remember this because my dad had pulled a reflex hammer from his old medical kit and done the same thing to us. The longer Stingley lay on the chalked grass, the more ashamed I grew. I knew, even then, that part of my attraction to football was the thrill of such violent transactions.

I can still see that hit. Stingley lowers his head just before impact. Tatum's shoulder pad strikes his helmet. What you don't see, what's safely hidden away under the armor, is how this impact compresses Stingley's spinal cord and fractures his fourth and fifth cervical vertebrae. Tatum and his teammates stride away from Stingley's grotesquely bent body with no apparent remorse.

What I remember most of all is the fear that dogged me in the days afterward, as it became clear that a star player had been rendered a quadriplegic on national TV: surely the game of football would now be outlawed.

Two years later, a congressional sub-committee did call Stingley to testify about a proposed bill to limit excessive violence in pro sports. But that measure, like other previous efforts, proved ceremonial. Instead, the Patriots gave Stingley a desk job and honored him in the manner of a war hero. Tatum, who was neither flagged nor fined for the hit, continued to terrorize opposing players. The NFL juggernaut rolled on. And I kept right on watching.

• • •

I spent most of my youth playing soccer. I was lucky enough to witness the first heyday of the pro game in this country. We lived twenty minutes from one of its marquee franchises, the San Jose Earthquakes. So why didn't I watch soccer instead? Why did I gravitate towards football? Why did I take up with the Raiders and remain loyal to them even after their rebel mystique had curdled?

I've argued above that the game of football is simply more gripping as a spectacle, a more faithful reenactment of our fundamental athletic impulses. But if we're going to be honest about all this, then we should specify what when we say "impulses," we're not just talking about the frolicking verbs—run, leap, catch—but the delight that boys (and later men) take in tackling and pounding and hurting.

And I should talk, too, a little more about the family in which I grew up. My parents met in medical school and later established private practices. They were politically active on the left. They made homemade jam and bread and candles. They read novels and performed Lieder as a duet, my father singing in German while my mother accompanied him on piano. They were gentle souls with three well-behaved sons who earned good grades. That was the public version of our family.

The private version was troubled. There was a lot of anger in our home and very little corresponding mercy. As I see it now, my folks had too many children too quickly—Dave was barely two when my twin Mike and I arrived. They felt overrun in ways that I, as a parent of three young children, am only beginning to comprehend.

My folks worked hard to connect with us individually. My dad, for example, coached my soccer team for years. But he and Mom also had ambitions of their own. And none of us boys, to be blunt, felt entirely secure in their love. We desperately wanted more attention, but this desperation frightened us, so we strangled it into silence. Rather than entreat our parents, we froze them out. It was how we punished them. We turned our brotherhood into a furious little fortress.

We sought to humiliate and injure one another constantly. I took a perverse pride in the fact that both of my brothers broke their hands in fights with me. One afternoon in high school I arrived home to find my brother Mike stomping around with a carving knife. Dave had stabbed him in the thigh with a fork and now he wanted revenge.

Beneath all the fury, we felt tremendous fear and despair. Later in life these emotions would bubble up through the cracks and swallow each of us, but back then we remained loyal to our chosen omertà. To reveal any weakness, to ask for comfort or love, was forbidden.

We all dealt with the pressure in different ways. My older brother maniacally pursued hobbies. My twin brother withdrew into himself. I watched football. In a home swirling with chaotic rage, it soothed me to see aggression granted a coherent, even heroic, context.

• • •

I'm setting all this out to explain why, even after watching a man get crippled, my devotion to the sport never wavered. My dad may have felt the same way, because I don't recall that we ever talked about the Stingley incident. We must have been content to write it off as a freak accident. We had that luxury back then.

We don't anymore.

Over the past few years, a growing body of medical research has confirmed that football can cause traumatic injury to the brain, not as a rare and unintended consequence, but as a routine byproduct of how the game is played. The central concern among doctors is no longer catastrophic injuries—concussions that result from big collisions—but the incremental (and therefore largely invisible) damage done by numerous sub-concussive hits.

A study commissioned by the NFL determined that recently retired pros (ages thirty to forty-nine) are nineteen times more likely to suffer from brain-trauma-related illness than—what's the right word here?—noncombatants. Given that aging stars don't want to be seen as disabled, they tend to downplay or even hide their infirmities. The numbers are likely higher.

Players may die younger, too. "Whereas white males live to 78 years and African-American males live to approximately 70 years, it appears that professional football players in both the United States and Canada have life expectancies in the mid to late 50s," according to Dr. Lee Nadler, the dean for Clinical and Translational Research at Harvard Medical School. Some researchers have claimed life expectancy for players is around fifty-five years of age.

NFL officials have sought to rebut these claims by trumpeting a 2012 study conducted by the National Institute for Occupational Safety and Health. It tallied death rates among more than 3,400 former players and concluded that they enjoy greater longevity.

But this approach, as any actuary would tell you, is inherently flawed, because the average age of death among men in the general population factors in those who die as children or young adults, as well as the poor, sickly, and undernourished. Oh, and smokers. The proper control for NFL players would be a cohort of super-fit, affluent, college-educated men. The study also tracked subjects who turned pro between 1959 and 1988, an era when players were much smaller. Until a sound longitudinal study is conducted, no one can say for sure how playing football effects mortality.

What has become increasingly obvious is that numerous NFL players incur brain damage. Doctors have autopsied the brains of dozens of former pros such as Junior Seau, Mike Webster, and Dave Duerson, and confirmed that they suffered from a form of dementia called Chronic Traumatic Encephalopathy (CTE). Like Seau, Duerson, an All-Pro safety, shot himself in the chest. Before taking his life, he sent his family a text message requesting that his brain be used for research.

A new crop of retired stars is just beginning to report

symptoms. Brett Favre, among the most heralded quarterbacks of the past two decades, shocked fans when he confessed to memory lapses last year. "I don't remember my daughter playing soccer one summer," Favre said. "So that's a little bit scary to me. For the first time in forty-four years, that put a little fear in me."

Terry Bradshaw was so concerned about his faculties that he sought diagnostic help five years ago. "I couldn't focus and remember things, and I was dealing with depression," the sixty-five-year-old Hall of Famer recounted. "I got tested to see what condition my brain is in. And it's not in real good shape."

Running back Tony Dorsett received the same news last year. At fifty-nine, he had been living with bouts of depression and memory loss. In a tearful television interview, he admitted he gets lost driving his daughters to their sports games. "It's painful, man, for my daughters to say they're scared of me . . . I've thought about crazy stuff, sort of like, 'Why do I need to continue going through this?' I'm too smart of a person, I like to think, to take my life, but it's crossed my mind."

Once again, nobody can say for sure what the prevalence rate of CTE is in active NFL players. The diagnostic tools don't exist yet. Doctors have yet to determine how factors such as drug use or genetic disposition might contribute to the brain damage they're seeing. And the sample group is admittedly skewed—former players whose families have submitted their brains for examination. But the numbers are stark. As of March, neuropathologists at the NFL's designated brain bank had examined fifty-five former football players. All but two showed signs of CTE. Already, the disease has been identified in the brains of deceased college players and even one high schooler.

The first wave of media coverage, two decades ago, focused narrowly on the impact of concussions. As doctors gathered more data, and shifted focus to the risks posed by the smaller collisions that occur every single play, the story evolved from a practical question—how to minimize big hits?—to an existential crisis.

It's useful to recall here the manner in which the public outcry over violence reshaped football a century ago. Back then, the President of the United States felt duty-bound to help speed reforms. The game was killing and maiming college and high school players. It was a moral problem.

The moment football became a business, violence was no longer just a moral problem. It was a money problem.

This, of course, is the big dance of capitalism: how to keep morality from gumming up the gears of profit, how to convince people to make bad decisions without seeing them as bad. We have whole industries devoted to this voodoo, the dark arts of advertising, marketing, public relations, lobbying. Every day, an army of clever men and women are devising new ways to get us to enjoy tobacco and animal flesh and petroleum and corn syrup without suffering the harsh aftertaste of guilt, without dwelling on the ethical costs of these pleasures. Oftentimes, you will hear some academic type marvel at the American capacity for self-delusion. Here's our secret: we're soaking in it.

I mention all this not just to get my socialist jollies, but to emphasize the larger system within which modern football operates. From the perspective of its governing body, the NFL, the game is a multi-billion-dollar product. And those of us who love it are not innocent *fans* rooting for our teams to prevail. We're *consumers*. Our money and attention are what subsidize the game.

This is true of all pro sports. But it's especially true of football. Consider this factoid. In 1948, nearly nine-tenths of the revenue earned by the NFL's best team, the Philadelphia Eagles, came from ticket sales. The share from radio and TV rights was 3 percent. Hardcore fans kept the league afloat, the ones who braved stadiums so cold that players sat bundled in hay to keep warm on the sidelines.

This season, the NFL will receive $5 billion in TV rights alone, nearly half its total revenue, and three times more than Major League Baseball earns. This money is generated by the tens of millions of casual fans engaged in what we might call "passive consumption" (i.e., watching a game on your couch while inhaling Cheetos).

But the league's ascendance has had unintended consequences. Stars now qualify as national celebrities, and their physical deterioration is front-page news. Television coverage renders each game as both epic and personal. Back in the seventies, the camera angles were limited and the images often grainy. The players remained obscure under their bulky exoskeletons, more like superheroes than human beings. Today, we see the game in high-def. Slow motion replays show us the unnatural angle of a broken ankle, and a quarterback's contorted face at the precise moment he is concussed. We hear the impact thanks to tiny microphones affixed to player's uniforms. It's gotten harder and harder for even casual fans to deny the cruelty of the game.

The standard rationalization hauled out at this point is that the NFL will clean up the game. As fans, we want to believe that league officials will choose the righteous path over the profitable one. This is nonsense and always has been.

From the beginning, the NFL has sought to obscure the most disturbing aspects of the game. This is why Bertie Bell, the first great commissioner of the NFL, wrote a stipulation into the contracts the league signed with TV networks prohibiting them from showing injuries or fights. "In the matter of television and radio we are doing a job for the public," he explained, "a job of showing them the best football in the world." In a more candid moment, Bell explained the appeal of the sport this way: "You knock my brains out this Sunday and I knock your brains out the next time we meet."

So football's guardians have always tried to walk this absurd line, between selling violence and disavowing it. The best way to gauge how league officials will respond to safety concerns is to consider what they have done thus far.

The first commissioner to issue a public statement on concussions was Paul Tagliabue, who succeeded Pete Rozelle in 1989. His statement: "On concussions, I think this is one of those pack journalism issues, frankly. The problem is a journalist issue." He cited steroids, drinking, and other injuries as more pressing matters.

Having served as the league's lead counsel before becoming commissioner, Tagliabue eventually adopted the same activist strategy employed by the tobacco industry. He sought to shape public debate by flooding the market with junk science. The NFL created a "research body" called the Mild Traumatic Brain Injury Committee. (If you believe, as I do, that language is essentially an instrument of truth, we might pause here a moment to linger upon the spooky propagandistic frisson produced by the juxtaposition of those two words: *mild, traumatic*.)

Tagliabue chose a man named Elliot Pellman to chair the committee. Pellman was a rheumatologist with no experience in brain research. He worked for the New York Jets and was Tagliabue's personal physician.

Members of the committee published sixteen papers in a medical journal called *Neurosurgery*, whose editor-in-chief was a consultant to the New York Giants. These papers invariably reached the same conclusion: NFL players were, if not impervious to brain injury, unlikely to suffer long-term effects. The authors, many of whom had worked in and around football for years, seemed at times almost touchingly naive about the fundamental nature of the game. ("Professional football players do not sustain frequent repetitive blows to the brain on a regular basis.") A number of these papers found a home in *Neurosurgery* only after being rejected by other editors and peer reviewers. Some were later repudiated by their own authors. Still, the committee provided crucial cover for Tagliabue. Every time some pesky reporter brought up concussions, he could point to the MTBI and its reams of exculpatory data.

The problem was that the number of former players showing signs of cognitive damage kept growing. They also began committing suicide in rather flamboyant ways. Steelers lineman Terry Long drank anti-freeze. His teammate Justin Strzelczyk led police on a high-speed chase before crashing into a tank truck at 90 mph. Long was forty-five, Strzelczyk thirty-six.

By the mid-2000s, a group of neurologists unaffiliated with the NFL had begun examining deceased players and finding incontrovertible evidence of brain damage that explained the disturbing symptoms of dementia reported by family members. In 2007, new commissioner Roger Goodell listened to a number of these doctors present their findings at a conference he convened on brain injuries.

His public response subtly undermined the link between football and brain damage. "I'm not a doctor, but you have to look at their entire medical history," he said. "To look at something that is isolated without looking at their entire medical history I think is irresponsible." The league also released a carefully worded pamphlet whose ostensible purpose was to inform players of the risks associated with concussions: "Current research with professional athletes has not shown that having more than one or two concussions leads to permanent problems if each injury is managed properly ... Research is currently underway to determine if there are any long-term effects of concussions in NFL athletes."

The league had entered its official Obfuscation Phase.

It didn't last long. Two years later, an NFL spokesman told a reporter this: "It's quite obvious from the medical research that's been done that concussions can lead to long-term problems." By this time, larger media outlets—*The New York Times* and *PBS* in particular—had begun piecing together the NFL's systematic cover-up. Players had begun to speak out and to consider legal remedy.

In 2011, a former Atlanta Falcons safety named Ray Easterling sued the NFL, an action eventually joined by more than 4,500 other former players. The suit accuses the NFL not only of negligence but fraud, a "concerted effort of deception and denial" that includes "industry-funded and falsified research."

In 2013, the NFL agreed to pay a settlement of $765 million, along with an estimated $200 million in legal fees. The presiding judge deemed this sum insufficient to cover the anticipated medical costs of the 20,000 players who eventually may qualify for payment.

Anybody with even a rudimentary sense of how corporations regard liability will understand why the NFL is so eager to make a deal. First, a settlement would guarantee that league officials never have to answer questions under oath regarding what they knew, and when, about the link between football and brain damage. Second, they would avoid the discovery phase, which would make public the grisly medical histories of former players. Presumably, some of these players and their family members would testify. It would be a public relations disaster.

And that's what matters, in the end, to NFL officials, and what makes their conduct so transparent. Roger Goodell and the men who work for him are not stupid. They've looked at the mountain of medical data and come to the same reluctant conclusion that Big Coal and Big Meat did decades ago. The business they run is unsafe for their workers.

The moral decision in this situation isn't very complicated: you stop playing the game until you learn more. You explain the dangers to your players (and the public) and you apologize for gambling with their health.

Goodell has made business decisions. He's done just enough—purged the deniers, tweaked the rules, funded research—to allow us fans to pretend that the league gives a damn. He's placed his faith in our capacity for self-delusion.

The second big rationalization in the NFL Fan Survival Kit is that players knowingly choose to incur the game's risks and are paid for doing so. You hear this line all the time on sports talk radio, often in that pitched, contemptuous tone characteristic of men who resent moral contemplation.

Okay. Let's start with the issue of what constitutes informed consent. Here's what seems fair: On NFL Draft Day, Roger Goodell can call the number one draft pick to the stage and give him his jersey and hat. But the commish will also have to hand the kid a waiver, the text of which would be printed on-screen:

> *I, _____, the undersigned, am aware that the average age of death of an NFL player is, according to some researchers, up to two decades shorter than normal life expectancy. Furthermore, I recognize that playing in the League, even in the absence of formally diagnosed concussions, may cause brain damage leading to the loss of cognitive function, depression, disorientation, and suicidal ideation.*

A copy of this waiver will be distributed to the draftee's family. They will then be required to watch a brief video of former players, such as the late Pittsburgh Steeler Mike Webster, describing—or attempting to describe—what life is like with CTE. Then the player and his family will be given a week to consider the matter.

That would be informed consent.

Most of those kids would sign. They would sign not just because they're twenty years old and believe they're bulletproof, but because their talent for football is the single attribute upon which they have been judged for most of their lives. Football isn't just what they do. It's who they are.

NFL players are members of an elite fraternity that knowingly places self-sacrifice, valor, and machismo above medical commonsense. Football is the one major American sport that selects specifically for the ability to inflict and absorb physical pain. (We don't judge baseball or basketball players on how well they can take a hit.) The ultimate badge of honor for a pro football player is not that he play *fair* or that he play *hard* but that he play *hurt*.

In January of 2014, ESPN asked 320 NFL players, anonymously, if they would play in the Super Bowl with a concussion. Eighty-five percent said yes. More recently, a linebacker for the Jacksonville Jaguars named Russell Allen revealed the reason for his unexpected retirement: he suffered a *stroke* after being hit during a game last year. Allen refused to leave the game or inform medical personnel because he feared he might lose his starting job.

One of the more despicable arguments put forward by the MBTI committee was that the rigors of football weeded out the weak. Those who made it to the pro level were less susceptible to concussions and quicker to recover from them. The proof of this claim was that so many players returned to the playing field so quickly after suffering concussions, which was a little like claiming that the dangers of black lung weren't that serious because so many coal miners returned to work after bouts of respiratory illness.

What an unbiased examination of the data suggests is

that concussions have been under-reported, under-diagnosed, and under-treated for decades. When doctors describe symptoms to an older player—dizziness, seeing stars—they often identify these as routine. The linebacker Bill Romanowski, by all accounts one of the nastiest players in league history, estimated that by these standards he'd suffered five hundred or more concussions during his career. "I saw stars every day for sixteen years. I saw stars in college." He was diagnosed with twenty concussions.

The NFL's research wasn't gauging the resilience of players' brains, but the toxic convergence of its own reckless cupidity with the macho culture that prevails among its employees.

What happens to a player who rejects this culture?

Consider the case of Ted Johnson. During his ten-year career, the hard-hitting linebacker helped the Patriots win three Super Bowls. In 2002, he suffered a concussion and briefly blacked out during a pre-season game. He returned to practice four days later, expecting he would wear a red jersey for "minimal contact." A blue "full contact" jersey was hanging in his locker. Johnson confronted a trainer, who told him there had been a mistake, that he wasn't cleared for contact. Johnson put on the red jersey. Out on the practice field, as the team prepared for a contact drill, an assistant trainer brought him a blue jersey. Coach Bill Belichick had directed him to do so. Johnson was incensed.

Here's where things get truly messed up.

Johnson put the jersey on anyway. Almost immediately, he suffered a second concussion and was rushed to the hospital. When he confronted Belichick privately, Johnson says the coach admitted that he'd screwed up and apologized to him.

Belichick's public response to the incident was considerably different: "If Ted felt so strongly that he didn't feel he was ready to practice with us, he should have told me."

This is part of what makes Bill Belichick a great coach. He knows how to "get the most out of his players," which is a kinder way of saying that he knows how to manipulate them. He knows that a tough guy like Johnson would rather risk his health than risk losing face by refusing to put on that blue jersey. "They weren't going to beat me," is how Johnson put it.

Instead, Belichick got Johnson to beat himself.

Johnson played three more seasons for the Patriots. He estimates that he suffered half a dozen more concussions, though he reported only one of them because he wanted to avoid being labeled soft. He was already suffering from symptoms of neurological damage, which have worsened.

If you follow football, especially in New England, you hear a lot of talk about the so-called "Patriot way," a dignified, stoic approach to the game. One of its central tenets is extreme secrecy when it comes to injuries. And yet here is how one team official summed up Johnson's medical condition to a *Boston Globe* reporter: "Ted Johnson is a very sick young man. We've been aware of the emotional issues he's had for years. You can't blame all of his behavior on concussions."

The Patriot Way: When a player receives serial brain traumas trying to honor your code, suggest in print that he is mentally ill.

Of course, it's easy to blame ruthless coaches and venal owners and foolhardy players, and much harder for us to see our own role in all this.

Most football players begin life with limited socioeconomic options. They may love football for its inherent virtues. But they also quickly come to see the game as a path to glory and riches. These rewards aren't inherent. They arise from a culture of fandom that views players as valuable only so long as they can perform.

We might pay lip service to health issues, but we're much less forgiving when the injury report comes out. Scroll through the Internet message boards, or listen to the provocateurs on sports talk radio. A frequently hurt player is not to be pitied, but suspected. In these kangaroo courts, "injury prone" has become synonymous with cowardly or weak-willed. The explosion in steroid use is partly a response to this mindset. The drugs help speed recovery from injuries.

Then again, according to a lawsuit filed in May, scores of ex-players were fed pain pills by team doctors and trainers—the pills were "handed out to us like candy," in the words of one retired lineman—and pressured to soldier on despite severe injuries. One of the named plaintiffs (there are more than five hundred in all), former Pro Bowl quarterback Jim

McMahon, claims he incurred a broken neck and ankle during his career, never received proper diagnoses, and played through both. Like other former players, McMahon wound up addicted to painkillers, and now suffers from the early stages of dementia.

We worship players for bravery and excoriate them for vulnerability because we wish to see masculine ideals on display. But I think here also of Cicero, who speculated that the loathing for timid gladiators wasn't a function of their diminished entertainment value but the fact that they forced spectators to confront the profound heartlessness of the games.

If you want to know what the current state of the research is on NFL players and brain damage, one of the best people on earth to consult is Dr. Ann McKee, co-director of the Center for the Study of Traumatic Encephalopathy at Boston University and chief neuropathologist for the National Veterans Affairs ALS Brain Bank in Bedford, MA. McKee is the person who cuts up the brains of former players and determines if they have CTE. Because so many brains have been coming in recently, and because (as her titles suggest) she is a very busy person, she is perpetually "about thirty brains behind."

She believes the gravest threat to players comes from sub-concussive hits, which the NFL's safety rules and concussion protocols won't prevent. The next milestone, McKee predicts, will be when doctors can measure brain injuries incurred during play, and brain disease in living players. "That will be the defining moment, the one that rewrites the book," she says. "I don't think we're that far away." She foresees a day when players entering the NFL will receive a risk assessment for brain damage based on factors such as genetic disposition, the number of years played, position, etc.

The introduction of such innovations would erode the haze of medical uncertainty that has long insulated the league and us fans. Imagine what would happen if word leaked that the top draft choice in 2017 stood a 25 percent chance of incurring brain damage five years into his career? Or if he was revealed to have incipient CTE? Or if fans had to confront not just replays of a superstar being knocked insensate, but a CAT scan showing the damage to his frontal lobes?

McKee is sometimes miscast as the bête noir of the NFL, because she was among the most visible early authorities on CTE. In fact, league executives dismissed her research for years. They've since adopted a kind of keep-your-enemies-closer approach by designating her lab as the league's "preferred" brain bank, and granting her millions in funding.

McKee is also, helpfully, an outspoken fan of the game. Her desk is surrounded by hundreds of slides of brain slices dyed to show areas with a buildup of tau, the cell-strangling protein symptomatic of CTE. Precariously balanced atop one stack of slides is a bobblehead doll of Aaron Rodgers, the quarterback of her Green Bay Packers.

McKee told me if she were a boy she would have played

football, and that she wanted her son to play. "When he got to high school, his dad didn't want him to play because it was too dangerous. I said, 'You've got to be kidding me.' It was horrifying to me!" McKee laughed. "So he played soccer."

I asked McKee how she justifies watching the game, knowing its dangers so intimately. "I don't know," she said. "I don't know where I am. I think it's a really important question. I have, like, these two faces. Right now they're pretty separate. I do watch a lot of football on Sunday."

In the morgue, a small, frigid room thick with the smell of preserving fluid, McKee lifted the lid of a white plastic bucket. Inside was a brain covered with splotches of dark crimson. "That's a suicide," explained her colleague, Dr. Victor Alvarez. McKee selected another brain and set it down on her cutting board. It looked like a small, discolored ham. She began slicing it up with a long scalpel.

Most of the brains McKee examines belong to veterans, not athletes. But the second brain she chose was a young female rugby player who had suffered a concussion, then continued to play. After a second impact, she suffered massive swelling of the brain and died. High school athletes are especially susceptible to so-called "second-impact syndrome."

I was there to talk to McKee about CTE, but the conversation between her and Alvarez and a young assistant named Brian quickly turned to the Super Bowl, which had been played a few weeks earlier.

Brian was a fan of the Denver Broncos, who had been routed. "After the first quarter, I just wanted it to be an entertaining game!" he said, carefully sliding brain slices into small plastic cases.

"After the first series!" said Alvarez, a Buffalo Bills fan.

At a certain point, I outed myself as a Raiders partisan, and we were off to the races.

It was an odd situation—actually *surreal* is closer to the mark. Even as McKee was dissecting this girl's hippocampus and amygdala and her delicate spinal cord, we were gabbing about football.

Before I left, McKee showed me two large color prints that hung in the hallway outside her office. One showed the brain of an eighteen-year-old football player with the brown spotting that signifies the onset of CTE. The other was a photo of a brain with two ghastly gouges in its frontal lobes, a lobotomy as they were conducted in the years after World War I.

A psychiatrist named Walter Freeman performed nearly 3,500 lobotomies, many of them by pressing an icepick through the corner of the eye socket and into the patient's brain. The procedure was sometimes used to treat victims of shell shock. The press hailed Freeman as a miracle worker. Only years later were his methods debunked. McKee marveled at the public acceptance of such barbarism, and I said, only half joking, that maybe decades from now the public will recoil at the thought that we ever watched a game that could permanently harm a teenager's brain.

"I've started to think it's impossible to change the NFL,"

McKee said. "People think none of this work will change the NFL."

She seemed completely blind to the irony hanging right in front of her. The ultimate agents of social change aren't researchers like her, but individual fans (like her) who confront the moral meaning of the research, who make the connection between the damaged brains—such as those McKee dissects—and their own behavior.

4

THIS EAGER VIOLENCE OF THE HEART

No one's saying it's easy. I've spent years trying to quit football, trying to view the game as a childish retreat from the world's real crises, a callous endorsement of authoritarian thinking, and so forth. During my post-collegiate Diaspora, I spent years wandering from one city to the next, searching, it seems to me now, mostly for a TV upon which I could watch the Raiders.

In Greensboro, North Carolina, where I arrived in the mid-nineties to become a writer and alienate everyone on earth, I hiked up to campus every Sunday looking for an empty student lounge. The Raiders themselves were never on. Still, I'd stand there for three hours watching teams I didn't even like, games that meant nothing in my grid of devotion, refusing to sit because I needed to believe I was going to be there for just a few minutes.

What kept me hooked was the limbic tingle familiar to any football fan, the sense that I was watching an event that *mattered*. The speed and scale of the game, the noise of the crowd, the grandiloquent narration and caffeinated camera angles—all these signaled a heightened quality of attention.

The players dashed about, their bodies lit in a kind of bright funnel of consequence.

A few years later I moved to Somerville, Mass, where I located a vast bacterial sports bar called the Good Times Emporium that catered to sickos like me. Imagine the wish complex of a thirteen-year-old boy detonated inside an airplane hanger: batting cages, bumper cars, paintball. They broadcast games at full-volume on giant washed-out screens, under which labored beautiful sullen barmaids with stretch marks and tattoos.

Every Sunday in autumn, I drove there to watch my team and to curse softly into my chicken wings. Because Good Times showed every NFL game, guys would show up in team jerseys and share pitchers of beer and roar together at the big plays and bellow at the injustices. We all understood the brazen con to which we were a party, that our primitive loyalties defined us as marks, that our favorite player might be gone by next year, or next week, that some gilded owner, if so inclined by market forces, would happily ship our entire team to a new city, that we were, objectively speaking, cheering for bright laundry.

Sometimes, during commercials, I would gaze around that bar, at the other men gazing upon their teams, the abject gleam in their eyes. In those moments I could see the tender truth nestled within each of us. We weren't rooting for our teams. We were rooting for ourselves.

• • •

Eventually, I got to recognize my fellow Raiders lifers. There were only four of us. We'd sit at separate tables and howl complaints, exchange looks of misery or the rare awkward high five. When the game was over, or we'd given up on the Raiders coming back, we'd leave without saying goodbye. The whole interaction felt illicit, intimate then shockingly hollow, like anonymous sex.

I told no one—not even close friends—about these excursions. They seemed unworthy of the literary artist I was striving, and failing, to become. But those afternoons were the central emotional events of my life. How else can I explain the way my hands would tremble in the parking lot? How my heart hammered the moment I saw the lovely silver and black of the Raiders' uniforms? After a tough loss, I would sit in my car and replay the fatal moments in my head until my fool heart ached.

There are all sorts of laudable reasons people watch sports, and football in particular. We wish to reconnect to the unscripted physical pleasures of childhood. We wish for moral structure in a world that feels chaotic, a chance to scratch the inborn itch for tribal affiliation. Sports allow men, in particular, a common language by which to converse.

When we root for a team, the conscious desire is to see them win, to bask in reflected glory. But the unconscious function of fandom is, I think, just the opposite. It's a form of surrender to our essential helplessness in the universal order.

In an age of scientific assurance, people still yearn for spiritual struggle. Fandom allows us to fire our faith in the forge of loss. Because our teams inevitably do lose. And this experience forms the bedrock of our identification.

Backing a team helps Americans, in particular, contend with the unease of living in the most competitive society on earth, a society in which we're *socialized* to feel like losers. That's the special sauce that capitalism puts on the burgers. It's how you turn citizens into efficient workers and consumers. You convince them that they are forever falling behind. Losing time. Losing money. Losing status. Losing hair. Losing potency. Losing the edge. We feel that we're losing all the time, simply by failing to win it all. We squander our talents, we mismanage the clock, we choke in the clutch. Our teams enact public dramas that we experience as struggles to transcend our own private defects.

We need look no further for evidence than to the proliferation of sports talk radio. Anyone who's listened to this format will tell you that nothing lights up the phone lines like a crushing loss. And what one hears in the callers' voices, beneath the bluster, is actually quite moving: an effort to preserve belief amid the tribulation of defeat.

I'm afraid that brings us back to the Raiders, and to the single play I have thought about more over the past decade than, for instance, the births of my children. (Please know that I am as disgusted with myself as you are right now.)

In January of 2002, the Raiders flew east to face the Patriots in a playoff game. I had been in Somerville a few years by then, and my friend Zach had stupidly agreed to let me watch the game at his place. I can still remember the color of the sky that morning, the dense gunmetal of a looming storm. By game time, huge, Hollywood-styled snowflakes were twirling down. They blotted out the yard markers and made traction nearly impossible, which lent the game a slapstick air.

The Raiders dominated, but the Patriots rallied late, led by a second-year quarterback named Tom Brady. Down three points with two minutes left, he dropped back to pass and found his receivers blanketed.

If I close my eyes I can still see Brady there, hopping about in the snow like a sparrow. He cocks his right arm as if to pass, thinks better of it, then pulls the ball down and pats it with his left hand. At this precise moment, Raiders cornerback Charles Woodson, deployed on an impeccably executed blitz, crashes into Brady and rakes away the ball. The ball lands in the snow, where it sits for an excruciating half-second. It is one of those enthralling moments, unique to football, where nobody knows what the hell is going on. At last, Raiders middle linebacker Greg Biekert falls on the ball. The Raiders can now run out the clock. The game is over.

I rose out of my chair and made animal sounds. Then I turned to Zach and said something gracious, how the Pats had played a good game, the kind of thing I can summon only when my team has won. Zach was still watching the TV.

Zach was still watching the TV because the referee had

announced that the play would be reviewed. Two minutes later, the referee clicked on his mic and explained that Brady was attempting to "tuck" the ball as he was stripped and was therefore, by some malicious metaphysical logic, still in the act of passing, rendering his fumble an incomplete pass. The Raiders never recovered from the shock. They lost the game in overtime. New England went on to win the Super Bowl.

If you were to plot the fortunes of NFL franchises on a graph—something I have come close to doing in dark moments—the Tuck Play would mark the spot where the Pats began their dynastic arc while the Raiders stumbled into disgrace. This play *should* have marked the spot on the map where my devotion waned.

Just the opposite happened. I spent the next hour (read: five years) trying to get Zach to admit that Brady had fumbled the ball. I argued with strangers, too. I nearly came to blows with a guy at my gym. And I tracked every phase of the Raiders' ensuing swoon, the carousel of inept coaches, the bungled draft picks, every senseless, drive-killing penalty.

A saner human being would have jumped ship years ago. Instead, I am that one sad asshole who quietly roots against the Pats every time they have a big playoff game—games, incidentally, that I often have to plead to watch at the homes of my friends, who hate having me there. But I am not a saner human being. Which is why I have watched the highlights of the Patriots losing their perfect 18–0 season to the Giants in Super Bowl XLII no fewer than twenty times.

• • •

There is no use in my attempting to justify this behavior. But the deranged patterns of our fandom, though they may manifest themselves in the here and now, took shape years ago. When I consider my earliest fervor for the Raiders, I don't think about the three Super Bowls they won. I think about the fact that they could never beat the Pittsburgh Steelers.

This is a direct result of growing up in the shadow of a domineering older brother who, mostly out of spite, rooted for the Steelers. I felt about the Raiders the way I felt about myself: that no matter what I achieved in the world, I would never vanquish Dave. And thus I spent the dim Decembers of my youth in the same state of grievance I would experience three decades later in New England.

The record books suggest that the Raiders beat the Steelers just as often as they lost. But what matters to a fan is the history your heart constructs. Long before the Tuck Play, I'd withstood the Immaculate Reception, in which Steelers running back Franco Harris plucked a deflected fourth-down pass off his shoe tops and galloped 43 yards for a touchdown with thirteen seconds left to knock the Raiders out of the playoffs. Cataclysm is my default setting as a fan.

I assumed that getting married and having kids would break my habit once and for all. But adult responsibilities have a way of sending us scurrying for the vestiges of our youth. Three seasons ago, I ordered a friend whom I was visiting to drive me thirty-five miles to a sports bar with satellite TV, all so I could watch the Raiders, finally within smelling distance of a playoff spot, destroy the 3–8 Miami Dolphins. After three quarters, Oakland trailed 34–0.

At such moments, sitting in a loud, corporate-themed sports bar in Greenville, South Carolina on the brink of tears, I am apt to reflect on the urtext of football freaks, Frederick Exley's novel *A Fan's Note.* "Whatever it was," he writes, "I gave myself up to the [New York] Giants utterly. The recompense I gained was the feeling of being alive."

It sounds romantic to be that abject. But the relationship Exley is describing is essentially vampiric. His hero looks to the Giants each Sunday to awaken him from the spiritual stupor of his life. That could be religion—or addiction.

"When I drank by myself, the liquor truly seemed like the one thing that gave me access to my true feelings," Caroline Knapp writes in *Drinking: A Love Story*, her searing account of alcoholism. It provided "an illusion of emotional authenticity which you can see as false only in retrospect." Reading these words, I thought about all the times I'd watched football alone, how much hope and sorrow had surged through me and how hollow I'd felt afterward, how hungover.

Knapp writes also about the camaraderie of drink, the way drunks will find cover by seeking out other drunks. This aspect of fandom may do the most, in the end, to insulate football from ethical scrutiny. The NFL, and the bloated media cult that feeds off of it, rely on us fans not to connect the dots. But to an even larger extent we rely on each other. There's safety in numbers.

As a writer living outside Boston, I tend to hang around with a bunch of highly educated smart alecks. But of all my male pals, there's exactly one who isn't conversant in football. The rest range from casual to fervent as fans. Here are the two most telling facts about this population.

Fact #1: They all admit to having moral qualms about watching football.

Fact #2: They all watch anyway.

Even the poets! My friend Dave is a Pittsburgh native who watched Tony Dorsett during his years at Pitt. He was so devastated to learn of Dorsett's cognitive decline that he lectured his college students about the tolls of football. He also confessed to me that he couldn't bring himself to take down the Terrible Towel hanging on the wall of his cubicle.

I've had a lot of difficult conversations with friends in the course of writing this book, none more so than with my neighbor Sean.

Sean is a former football player and what I like to call a fracture-level fan. Some months ago, he showed up at my house with a cast on his hand from accidentally punching a wooden bed railing during a game. (I myself have punched many wooden objects during games, always intentionally and never with sufficient force to break a bone.) It might be worth mentioning that Sean is six-four and 260 pounds. When I talked with him at the outset of this project, he looked at me for a few long seconds then said, in a quiet, imploring voice, "Please don't take this away from me."

For the past five years, Sean and I have sought refuge from the pressure cooker of family life. We have done this *not* by tearing out of our homes and jumping on the motorcycle Sean has been rebuilding for the past three years and gunning it down to Daytona Beach and guzzling enough tequila to participate in an ironic wet T-shirt contest for sad, middle-aged men and then blacking out—but instead by watching football games together. That's the "this" I assumed he meant.

But it turns out Sean's fandom is far more organic than mine. He grew up in semi-rural West Virginia, football country. He was a natural from early on, a kid with that rare combination of size, speed, and agility. Virtually everyone in his life expected him to become a football player, especially his father. When I asked him why he quit, he told me this story:

When he was about eleven years old, his team played a rival with the best running back in the league. It was Sean's role, as the star of the defense, to contain the kid. On one play, Sean met the running back just as he was about to burst through a gap. The running back lowered his head, in the same instinctual way Darryl Stingley had, and their helmets collided at full speed. The kid fell and lay motionless.

The kid's coaches, and later his parents, ran onto the field. Smelling salts didn't revive him. Eventually, an ambulance appeared. Sean was convinced he'd killed the boy. He began to cry. But what Sean remembered most vividly was how, right after the tackle, his teammates kept slapping his helmet, as if he'd just done the most heroic thing ever, which, in a purely football sense, he had. He also recalled trying to walk away from his teammates, because he didn't want them to see that he was crying. Even three decades later, recounting this episode shook up Sean.

The running back did not wind up paralyzed. That's not the point of the story. It was the tremendous anguish Sean felt over his power to harm another boy, and to be revered for this power. A burden heavy enough to make him walk away—despite his love of the game and his natural gifts.

Because of his size, Sean has spent the rest of his life having to tell people he doesn't play football. And even though he's now a respected digital archivist at M.I.T., with a beautiful wife and two children, there's still some core part of him that wishes he had played, that knows he squandered a shot at greatness. Football remains the unrequited love of his life.

And now here I was—his designated football buddy!—suggesting that even being a fan of the game was wrong. Don't we turn to football precisely to escape such complexities, to watch the miracle of supreme bodies at play, to pretend, however briefly, that life is just a fearless game?

Still, I can't help thinking about something else Sean told me, which was how, in the hours and days after he delivered his big hit, he kept asking the same question of his coaches: "I didn't do anything wrong, did I?"

5

"GET MONEY!" ON THREE

I was on an airplane watching television, which is not a statement that would have made sense even ten years ago, but there you go. Thank you, America. Among the suite of channels was the NFL Network, which I predict will soon be the world's most popular cable channel and will spawn a second and third channel, if it hasn't already. I wasn't supposed to be watching football, but they were showing the NFL Combine, where the league gathers top college prospects to put them through their paces. I couldn't resist.

The drill I happened to see was for defensive backs. They had to backpedal then whirl around and catch a ball fired at them at about 200 mph. Afterward, a gentleman named Peter Giunta, the secondary coach for the New York Giants, called the prospects together to give them an inspirational speech. Giunta was bald and intense. His rhetorical style fell somewhere between General Patton and Tony Soprano. "It is a privilege to play in the National Football League," he began. "It is not your *right* . . . You have to do the right things, not only on the field but off the field. They've done security checks on you, background checks. I don't wanna read about you in the papers. We live in a great country. We all have the power of choice."

He continued on this theme for several minutes. Then he called upon Bradley Roby, a projected first-rounder from Ohio State, to lead a final cheer. The players huddled up. "We all know why we're here," Roby barked. " 'Get money!' on three."

One, two, three. Get Money!

It is always refreshing when people are honest in this way. And it is particularly refreshing when it comes from the NFL, because there is so much horseshit swirling around regarding the economic forces that drive the game.

The most persistent myth about the NFL is that, because of its revenue sharing system, it is somehow socialist. To quote the writer Chuck Klosterman: "The reason the NFL is so dominant is because the NFL is basically Marxist."

Klosterman has written a lot of intelligent analysis of the NFL over the years. This is not a prime example.

As noted, NFL owners in large cities agreed to divide TV proceeds equally back in 1962, in part to create competitive balance on the field. That is not Marxism. It is, at best, a canny form of market manipulation. But the history is far more problematic. In fact, Pete Rozelle had signed a TV contract in 1960 on behalf of the entire league—a deal struck down by a federal court as a violation of antitrust law. Rozelle went to Washington, and lawmakers obediently passed the

Sports Broadcasting Act of 1961, which allowed the NFL and other leagues to circumvent those pesky antitrust rules and to sell TV rights, collectively, to the highest bidder. The law essentially made the NFL a legal monopoly.

But just as a thought experiment, let's pretend the NFL really *were* Marxist. Here's what that would mean. First, there would be no private ownership, and therefore no team owners. The teams, though they would represent different cities, would belong to the State. Employees would be paid according to the Marxist edict: *From each according to his ability, to each according to his need.* A top quarterback such as Peyton Manning would not be paid $18 million every season. He would be paid based on his needs, let's say $100,000 per year. The worker who laundered his jock strap, or the custodian who mopped the floors of his locker room might be paid just as much as Peyton Manning—perhaps more if they had greater needs, say, a lot of children or sick parents. Star athletes could still ostensibly earn huge sums in endorsement deals from private industry, though the league would have to decide whether these payments violated its Marxist tenets. Commissioner Goodell would not receive a compensation package of $42.2 million, as he did in 2012, nor would his deputies earn millions.

In fact, one of the most fascinating questions that arises from a truly Marxist NFL would be the question of what to do with the staggering profits, which would no longer be divvied up by a cabal of geriatric magnates or funneled to a pack of vainglorious athletes. We can safely assume that its operating costs would be a fraction of the nearly $10 billion the NFL is projected to earn this season. The balance—$9.5 billion?—would be available for redistribution to societal needs such as early education, medical and renewable energy research, intervention for at-risk populations. Fans would be in the strange position of justifying their support of pro football by pointing to all these good works.

A Marxist NFL, in which salaries were no longer grossly inflated by our blessed free market, might spur other felicitous outcomes as well. Players could choose to join clubs in the cities or states where they actually grew up. With obscene economic incentives removed, players and fans might experience the sport as a purer form of meritocracy. As with the NCAA basketball tournament, competition would hinge on team and regional pride rather than individual earning power. There would be no more parasitic entourages or predatory agents. And almost certainly, athletes would make more sensible decisions regarding their own health.

Do I realize this will never *ever* happen? That lawyers would descend from their penthouse aeries to sue the bejesus out of all parties? That the players themselves would flee the NFL in droves to join for-profit leagues, or form their own? That Rush Limbaugh's head would explode as he tried to process the concept of a "socially-conscious blood sport."

Yes. Which is my point.

The NFL is the opposite of Marxist. It is the epitome of

crony capitalism, a corporate oligarchy that has absorbed or crushed all potential competitors, that routinely extorts municipal and state governments, and openly flouts its tax obligations while remaining, in the words of *The Atlantic*'s Gregg Easterbrook, "walled off behind a moat of anti-trust exemptions."

The league's players are among the most specialized employees on earth. Every aspect of their job performance is filmed, analyzed, measured, and submitted to public scrutiny. Minute differences in efficiency translate into mind-boggling pay discrepancies. It is this ruthless workplace that compels so many players to play through pain, shoot up steroids, etc.

Much is made of the communal virtues imparted by football: sportsmanship, teamwork, self-sacrifice. But a genuine Marxist would note that these qualities are placed in the service of contests whose outcomes are irrelevant to the fate of the worker. Football is the ultimate bourgeois indulgence. Its civic function is to distract the proletariat from the aims of the revolution and to serve as a means of indoctrination into thought systems that are individualistic and materialist.

Think about it, folks. Last season, the Minnesota Vikings paid a man named Jared Allen more than a million dollars *per game* to maul opposing quarterbacks. The "market"—meaning us, the fans—has determined that Allen's value is roughly $18.5 million per year. The State of Minnesota pays an elementary school teacher an average of $38,000 per year. Paramedics make $42,000; cops, $28,000. That makes one quarterback mauler worth 474 elementary school teachers. Or 440 paramedics. Or 661 police officers.

Let us pause in astonishment and torment.

The closer you look, the worse it gets. Consider that in 2013, lawmakers in Minnesota voted to allot $506 million in taxpayer money to the Vikings to help them build a new stadium—despite facing a $1.1 billion state budget deficit. They did this because Vikings ownership had made noises about relocating the team, a tactic routinely used against politicians who live in terror of losing a franchise. The new stadium increased the value of the team by an estimated $200 million. The owners, who are multi-millionaires, pay $13 million per year to use the stadium, which sounds like a lot until you consider that they earn *hundreds of millions* in TV revenues, ticket sales, concessions, and parking. This helps explain why teachers and social workers get paid what they do in Minnesota.

Here's the totally nutso part: the Vikings' ownership actually *underperformed*. Based on research done by Judith Grant Long, a professor of urban planning at Harvard, taxpayers provide 70 percent of the capital cost of NFL stadiums, as well as footing the bill for "power, sewer services, other infrastructure, and stadium improvements."

The perfect example: Seven of every ten dollars spent to build CenturyLink Field in Seattle came from the taxpayers of Washington State, $390 million total. The owner, Paul Allen, pays the state $1 million per year in "rent" and collects most of the $200 million generated. If you are wondering how to become, like Allen, one of the richest humans on earth, negotiating such a lease would be a good start.

In New Orleans, taxpayers have bankrolled roughly a billion dollars to build then renovate the Superdome, which we are now supposed to call the Mercedes-Benz Superdome. Guess who gets nearly all the revenues generated by Saints games played in this building? If you guessed all those hard-working stiffs who paid a billion dollars, you would be wrong. If you guessed billionaire owner Tom Benson, you would be right. He also receives $6 million per annum from the state as an "inducement payment" to keep him from moving the team.

That's the same amount Cowboys owner Jerry Jones would pay each year in property taxes to Arlington, Texas, where his fancy new stadium is located. Except that Jones doesn't pay property taxes because, like many of his fellow plutocrats, he's cut a sweetheart deal with the local authorities.

In the old days, NFL owners were rich men who accepted the risk of losing money as the cost of doing business. Thanks to the popularity of the game, the NFL and its owners—with the collusion of politicians—have created what amounts to a risk-free business environment. According to Long's data, a dozen teams received more public money than they needed to build their facilities. Rather than going into debt, they turned a profit.

• • •

Let's take another big step backward.

Okay, so taxpayers have funded 70 percent of the construction costs of the stadiums in which NFL teams play, for which they receive a return of pennies on the dollar. But consider the economic impact if taxpayers were to receive 70 percent of the profits generated by those facilities: that is, a proportion equal to our investment. Given that the NFL is projected to earn in the neighborhood of $10 billion this season, that amounts to $7 billion from TV, tickets, parking, etc. (Again: no stadiums means no games.) Think about how much social *good* $7 billion would do in cities such as Detroit and Cleveland and St. Louis, where bright new stadiums rise above crumbling schools, closed factories, and condemned homes.

Or let's say, more conservatively, that cities demanded a 50 percent share of the profits as rent. Or simply demanded that the owners remit to the taxpayers the sum required to build and maintain these stadia. This would still represent hundreds of millions of dollars.

This is not some socialist "redistribution of wealth" scheme. It's not charity. That's Fox News math. This is asking an immensely profitable business to pay investors (taxpayers) our rightful dividend.

The traditional line put forward by boosters is that a sports franchise generates prestige and jobs and economic growth for a particular city. It would be more accurate to characterize teams as parasites on the local economy. They suck money from local tax bases then send the gigantic profits generated by these expenditures back to the league office for disbursement to the owners.

Think about how insane our cultural priorities are that we're allowing so much money to be siphoned from the public till and funneled directly into the private koi ponds of the nation's wealthiest families. That arrangement isn't even capitalist. It's feudal.

Please try to imagine, if you would, what other industry could perpetrate such financial chicanery and still be considered a model corporate citizen? Think about this the next time the NFL ballyhoos one of its PR charity giveaways.

This is not a matter of politics, by the way. Conservatives who rail against government debt and liberals who lament the decline of social services should be equally outraged. Better yet: they should recognize that their loyalty to the NFL is what makes this ongoing confidence game possible. We are the ones who give the league its tremendous leverage over politicians. We shouldn't be surprised that it uses this leverage. That's what capitalists do.

A relevant memory: A few years ago I traveled down to Miami, where I worked as a reporter during the early nineties. A friend was driving me around downtown when I noticed what looked like a large-scale demolition project.

"What's that?" I said.

My friend shook his head. "They're tearing down the arena," he said.

"The *Miami* Arena?" I said.

The arena had just gone up when I moved to town fifteen years earlier, as a home for the NBA's newest franchise, the Miami Heat. It had been built with public money, naturally. But that was okay, because the arena was going to be the savior of an impoverished area known as Overtown.

Now the building was being razed, a pink elephant that had cost taxpayers more than $50 million. It had diverted precious funds and political will from legitimate plans to economically develop Overtown, where, according to the most recent census figures, the per capita annual income is less than $15,000, and half of all children are living in poverty. Now, county officials were spending $210 million in public money on a new bayside arena for the Heat.

During my time in Miami, I had spoken briefly with one of the few dissenting voices, a county commissioner named Katy Sorenson, whose reaction to the Miami Arena plan I have never forgotten. Here is what she said:

> The real quality-of-life issues are jobs and job training and child care for people seeking job training. It's schools and health care and parks. It's about making sure people feel safe . . . Those are the things that will really make this a great county. Not an arena. This is about a bunch of spoiled, overfed, overpaid corporate giants who are having an arena built by taxpayers so that a bunch of spoiled, overfed, overpaid athletes can have a place to play.

And now there sat the Miami Arena, floating in a vast landscape of concrete and blight, as the demolition crews did their taxpayer-funded work. All I could think was: this is the story of modern America under the influence of sports. The carnival comes to town and everyone gets drunk on the spectacle and empties their pockets and by morning the carnies are gone and what you thought was an enchanted kingdom full of prizes is just a muddy field on the edge of town.

But that's not quite right, because fans form long-term relationships with their teams. The Browns started playing in Cleveland in 1945, for instance. They won eight championships in their first two decades and earned a zealous following. This did not stop owner Art Modell from announcing, in the middle of the 1995 season, that he was moving the team to Baltimore (itself abandoned by the Colts a dozen years earlier). Modell inked this deal the day *before* voters approved a plan that had been put on the ballot at his request to revamp Cleveland Municipal Stadium for $175 million. During the Browns' final home game, fans set fires in the stands, heaved rows of empty seats onto the field, and tore bathroom sinks from the walls.

But Modell was merely following the rules of the modern NFL cartel. By moving to a new city desperate for football he secured a brand new stadium worth $220 million—with taxpayers picking up $200 million of that tab—where the newly minted Baltimore Ravens could play, rent-free, for thirty seasons, with Modell keeping every cent from tickets, parking, naming rights, concessions, and the sale of 108 luxury boxes and 7,500 club seats. Modell used the proceeds from personal seat licenses—fans who pay for the *right* to buy tickets—to build a $15 million training facility and cover his moving and legal fees. (Spurned Cleveland fans filed more than one hundred lawsuits against him.) Within a few years, his team—purchased in 1961 for $3.9 million and valued at $163 million before departing Cleveland—was worth $600 million.

The same scenario was playing out all over the country, with owners securing eye-popping deals (and thus multiplying franchise value) by moving to new cities, or threatening to. Houston lost the Oilers to Nashville. St. Louis lost the Cards to Phoenix. Because of the insatiable market created by us fans—particularly in jilted cities—the NFL could also auction off the right to expansion teams, thus increasing the pool of potential civic suitors for owners to wield against their hometowns.

Franchise Free Agency, as it is sometimes called, is better understood as a highly public Ponzi scheme. The league pits cities and citizens against each other and sweeps up the profits. A Houston billionaire eventually paid the NFL a $700 million expansion fee to replace the Oilers, outbidding Los Angeles. The public chipped in $250 million for a new stadium.

And what about poor Cleveland? The NFL graciously bestowed the city an expansion team (franchise fee: a paltry $476 million) and lucky taxpayers shelled out almost $300 million to build them a new home. A fairytale ending, NFL style.

As for my Raiders, our late owner Al Davis—a man best described as Corleonish—made a career out of extorting the City of Oakland. He moved the team to Los Angeles from 1982 to 1994, and secured $220 million in stadium renovations to return to Oakland, plus a training facility, moving costs and, presumably, his weight in cannoli. While the city is still paying off those renovation bonds, the team pays $525,000 per year in rent.

I would be remiss if I failed to note one more fiscal oddity. The NFL—unlike the NBA and Major League Baseball—is tax-exempt. How did this happen?

Funny you should ask.

Back in 1966, when the league was hashing out a deal with Congress that would allow it to merge with the AFL, lobbyists managed to insert a provision into the tax code allowing "professional football leagues" to be granted not-for-profit status. All the NFL had to do was pledge not to schedule games on Friday nights or Saturdays, to avoid competing with high school and college games.

The tax exemption (501(c)6, for those keeping score at home) was originally intended for "business leagues, chambers of commerce, real-estate boards, or boards of trade"— local industry groups that welcome new members. I wish all of you good luck in your efforts to join the NFL.

This does not mean that the league's revenues are all untaxed. The NFL League Office distributes earnings to its member teams, which are for-profit entities and therefore should pay taxes. However, because owners have proven so adept at cutting deals to reduce their tax burdens, and because their records are private, no one knows what sort of tax rate owners pay on their profits. We can safely assume they do better at finding deductions than those of us who don't own NFL teams.

As not-for-profit organizations go, the NFL isn't exactly small-time. In addition to rent on their spacious Park Avenue offices, the league pays $60 million in executive salaries. Half of this sum goes to Commissioner Goodell.

Last year, Senator Tom Coburn, a conservative from Oklahoma, proposed legislation that would bar any sports league with profits exceeding $10 million annually from claiming tax-exempt status. Coburn has noted that NFL officials not only duck federal taxes but use their exempt status to avoid city and state taxes when they travel on league business, to the Super Bowl for instance.

Oh, one other key league expenditure: lobbying. The NFL pays $2 million per year for that.

Coburn's proposal has never been debated, let alone voted upon.

Hosts on sports talk radio will sometimes argue that fans shouldn't complain about the monstrous salaries athletes receive, because our support makes them possible. But the athletes are really just the public face of a much larger enterprise. We could call them pawns. A better analogy would be corner drug boys. They supply us our high and palm our cash. They run the risk while their employers, operating out of sight, collect most of the proceeds. Let's at least be honest about whom we're really enriching: the One Percent.

Most fans turn to football for idealistic reasons. We love being immersed in its gallant meritocracy. We want to believe the game is played primarily for honor, not money. But, as the game has morphed from a ragged outlier into a corporate juggernaut, we've evolved as fans, too. Think about how much time we spend these days obsessing over the economics of the game. Hardcore fans think as much about salary cap hits as corner blitzes. We crunch numbers and debate player valuation and second-guess every move management makes.

Is it any wonder fantasy football leagues have become so popular? The fantasy, after all, is one of ownership, of competing to see who can best manage human capital. I spent two years in such a league. After a while I didn't really care which teams won anymore. I just wanted to score more points than everyone else. I was rooting for my own acumen.

With considerable regret, I must now ask you to take one final step backward, so as to ponder the NFL's long-range game plan.

In 2010, Roger Goodell (whose pay is based largely on

how much he can grow profits) announced that he hoped the NFL would reach revenues of $25 billion by 2027. This represents an increase of 250 percent over the next fourteen years. It would put the NFL on par with global Goliaths such as Nike and McDonalds, and exceed the entire GDP of more than a hundred countries.

Where do you think these additional monies are going to come from? They are going to come from you and me, in the form of more public subsidies for more palatial stadiums, and higher prices for tickets, parking, and all the rest.

In an era of DVRs and digital streaming, football games remain one of the few events some people (i.e., us addicts) insist on watching live. And we don't just tolerate the commercials during games, in the case of the Super Bowl we actually celebrate them. This has made NFL football, by far, the most valuable entertainment commodity in the world. And it's what makes the league's monopoly status so lucrative, according to John Vrooman, an economist at Vanderbilt University who has written extensively about the NFL's fiscal ploys.

League officials can negotiate all-or-nothing broadcast rights and advertising rates, and thus set prices much higher than individual teams in competition ever could. Those higher prices inevitably (and invisibly) get passed on to us consumers, who wind up paying more for cable TV and products.

Vrooman predicts the league will eventually limit access to games unless fans are willing to pay a premium. "The monopoly rule is to gouge half as many fans more than twice as much on everything," he says. League officials and owners insist they won't turn football into a luxury item. But that's exactly what they're doing right now by building all those corporate suites and broadcasting certain games exclusively on the NFL Network.

The tremendous value of these games is the reason Goodell—even in the face of a growing crisis over player health—is quietly pushing to increase the season from sixteen to eighteen games, and to expand the playoffs.

We fans can romanticize the game all we like, but Goodell and his bloodless syndicate deal in leverage and maximization. Here's how Brian Rolapp, the Chief Operating Officer of NFL Media, and the man tasked with making sure pro football dominates the digital age (he just brokered deals with Verizon, Twitter, and Microsoft) puts it: "We're really in the business of aggregating America around events and around our game. There are fewer and fewer places that can do that. If you can aggregate audiences, you are going to be more and more valuable."

How romantic.

Let us return, then, to that scene at the NFL Combine, to those defensive backs who have just finished their drill and heard that inspirational speech about the privilege of playing in the NFL and making the right decisions. "We all know why we're here," Bradley Roby shouts. " 'Get money!' on three."

It's easy for fans to dismiss a moment like this as reflective of some unfortunate "ghetto mentality." It becomes much more depressing to admit that Roby is parroting the guiding ethos of the NFL, and the private sector.

The truth is, I have a lot *more* respect for Roby. If you grew up amid the kind of deprivation that a lot of NFL prospects did, and football represented your one best chance to lift yourself and your loved ones out of poverty, why the hell wouldn't you want to get money?

It's a lot tougher for me to sympathize with mercenary executives and team owners who were born into affluence. Why must they squeeze every penny from their position of cultural power? Do they feel no shame in snatching taxpayer money they don't really need from impoverished communities? Is the acquisition of capital the only way they know how to keep score? At what point do we admit that the NFL's true economic function is to channel our desire for athletic heroism into an engine of nihilistic greed?

6

THE LOVE SONG OF RICHIE INCOGNITO

I once made the mistake of watching a football game with an Italian woman who was studying medieval gender roles, and with whom, rather unimaginatively, I hoped to have sex. It was the sort of mistake one makes in one's twenties, before one has developed a proper appreciation for the virtues of compartmentalization.

"They are spending most times hugging," Elena observed.

"Those are blocks," I said.

"Then at the end, they make a big pile on the ground and grind each other."

"There's no grinding."

"Then they spank the others on the behind. It's a gay ritual!"

"I don't think so," I said.

"But look. Before each time, the skinny one, the sex leader—"

"The *quarterback*—"

"He makes all the big boys bend over. Then he chooses his favorite and comes up behind the lucky one and makes a pantomime of sodomy."

"No," I said. "No no no. That's the snap. It's how the play starts. And the quarterback gets the ball from one guy, the center. It's not a choice. He can't just come up to, like, the tight end."

Elena looked at me for several complicated European seconds. "The *what*?"

Earlier this year, a University of Missouri football player named Michael Sam announced that he was gay. He'd never worked hard to hide who he was. He dated a man throughout college. He frequented a gay club in Columbia. He came out to his college teammates before his last season. Many of them already knew.

As a kid growing up in Texas, Sam watched one of his older brothers die from a gunshot wound. Two more of his seven siblings died, and two others were imprisoned. He was once maced by police officers who had come to his house to arrest a relative. He also lived, briefly, in his mother's car. These events probably helped Michael Sam put the issue of his sexual orientation into perspective.

In May the St. Louis Rams drafted the highly touted defensive end in the seventh round. If Sam makes the team, he will be the first openly gay player in NFL history. And thus his decision not to hide his sexual orientation—what we heterosexuals think of as *living*—became a huge story.

The underlying premise of this story was that the NFL might not be "ready" for an openly gay player. Reporters found sources to mouth the necessary misgivings. Anonymous team officials fretted that Sam's draft stock would drop because of the media distraction he might cause, to which they were naturally (and, again, anonymously) contributing.

It was one of those media narratives in which the alleged subject (*Michael Sam: Gay Guy in Shoulder Pads*) was much less interesting than the actual subject: *A Workplace Exists in America, Circa 2014, in Which the Prospect of Accommodating a Single Openly Gay Employee Is Enough to Induce Panic.*

In what other setting would this sort of bigotry be tolerated? The Armed Forces used to be an acceptable standby. At this point, we're down to outfits run by fundamentalist religious groups.

The logic seems to be that football is a domain of hyper-masculinity, a physical and psychological space where alpha males do battle. And gay men can't be alphas because they are fragile and frightened and weak, which is to say feminine.

And everyone knows (and curiously consents to the fact) that the assigned roles of the feminine in football remain safely locked in the pre-suffrage era. The two archetypes seen most commonly on television are cheerleaders and players' wives. Got that, ladies? You can either dance around on the sidelines as a half-naked sex object or sit in the stands cheering on your man. It remains unclear to me why so many women watch football, given how dismissive the game is of them.

But I'm more interested, for now, in the way a figure like

Sam exposes the neurotic sexual conflicts at the heart of football.

Here, for instance, is how a linebacker named Jonathan Vilma explained his concerns about having Sam as a team-mate: "Imagine if he's the guy next to me and, you know, I get dressed, naked, taking a shower, the whole nine, and it just so happens he looks at me. How am I supposed to respond?"

Vilma's point is that, unlike employees in other lines of work, he might have to be naked in front of Sam, which would make him feel uncomfortable. Fair enough.

But can I just ask: Why is Jonathan Vilma haunted by a fantasy *of his own devising* in which he is standing naked next to Michael Sam and being visually inspected by him, maybe even (gasp) admired? What is Vilma—a player so vicious that he was suspended for four games last season for attempting to injure opposing players—really afraid of here? That the simple act of a gay man looking at his naked body will call his own sexuality into question? That he'll catch gay cooties? That Sam will overpower him and force him to have gay sex? Why does Vilma imagine that he has to respond to Sam at all?

Before I go any further with this disquisition, let me confess that I get what Vilma was saying. And if you stripped away all my sensitivo politesse—or just plunked me in front of an NFL game with a bunch of soused buddies—I would cop to the same worry. That's why I feel comfortable speculating about Vilma's motives. We've got the same issues. Almost all straight men do. We're afraid of being gay, and that fear (whether we like it or not) contains an unconscious wish. Freud himself believed that we begin life with unfocused libidinal drives and that, though most of us settle into an orientation, we retain an attraction to both sexes.

For the record, if this isn't already clear, I grew up in a male-dominated home where insecurity and bullying and homoeroticism ran rampant. I dealt with my confusion by throwing myself into sports, as a player and fan. Like a lot of guys, I believed that being a jock, albeit an inept one, would vouchsafe my heterosexuality.

And yet it's also true that I found in the world of sports a way to sublimate my feelings of affection and desire for men. I did look at other guys in the locker room and I thought a lot about their bodies. I didn't fantasize about having sex with them, but I did envy the power and confidence they possessed and I wanted to be close to them. It got sloppy. I can remember my mother walking into my room one night only to discover, to her obvious distress, that I was giving a back massage to a shirtless friend. Another time, behind a locked door, two soccer buddies and I measured our erect cocks in anguished silence. That's a decent executive summary of my adolescence: endless dick measuring.

After his first year in college, my twin brother Mike told me he was gay. I was absolutely floored. I'd been harboring the suspicion that he was sleeping with my girlfriend. He had dated women in high school and been a standout on the swim and water polo teams. But I wonder now if my obsession with sports was in some ways a response to whatever part of me recognized Mike as gay. Later on, it would become clear that Mike tended to date African-American men. Was my fandom in some ways a coded expression of the same attraction?

My own view of sexuality at this point lines up with Kinsey. Our desires are a lot more fluid than we like to admit— a spectrum, not a duality. I like to joke that my friend Billy (who hates sports and dresses like the New Jersey equivalent of a peacock) is 23 percent gay. What I'm really saying is that I'm 23 percent gay. That's how it works with homophobia. It's just one big projection racket. Anybody who says he hates gay people is really saying he hates the secret gay parts of himself.

I believe there have always been people who are more sexually attracted to their own gender than the opposite gender, and the ones with the courage to admit to these impulses and act upon them get labeled gay. In the end, if you look at things objectively, it should make very little difference how people find sexual happiness. It's their business, just like your sex life is your business. Parts is parts.

Our sexual morality is almost entirely culturally determined. In the world of the Old Testament—a world defined by the patrilineal inheritance of land and the expansion of power by marriage—homosexuality mucked up the given order. So God told a story about how it was deviant. In ancient

Greece, grown men wooed and bedded teenage boys. The mightiest Greek soldier of all time, Achilles, loved his friend Patroklus more than any concubine. Nobody freaked.

Here in America, at the dawn of the third millennium AD, 60 percent of us support same-sex marriage. But there's still this huge undertow of masculinity anxiety. And the preserve where this anxiety finds its purest and most obvious expression is in the Athletic Industrial Complex, especially in the game of football.

No other major sport defines masculinity in such radical terms, as both violent and physically intimate. It is my own belief that the brutality of the game is what allows for such intimacy. Men purchase the right, through their valor, to love other men without experiencing shame. Football is a form of camouflage, a display of manliness so overt that the viewer never questions the game's subtle oddities.

And I suppose this brings us right to the main event, a document called *The Wells Report*, which was compiled, at the NFL's direction, after the starting left tackle for the Miami Dolphins, Jonathan Martin, left the team last October and checked into a nearby hospital for psychological treatment. He quit due to "persistent bullying." *The Wells Report* offers a rare peek inside the sanctum of an NFL locker room. It also presents a riveting and unintended saga of homoerotic turmoil.

The dramatis personae are mostly members of the

offensive line, a close-knit unit led by a charismatic veteran named Richie Incognito. The authors affirm that Incognito, along with fellow vets Mike Pouncey and John Jerry, engaged in "a pattern of harassment" toward Martin that went beyond the standard rookie hazing. Press reports focused on the racial epithets that Incognito, who is white, directed at Martin, who is African-American. Among the more poetic sobriquets: "half-nigger piece of shit," "shine box," "stinky Pakistani" and "darkness."

Incognito also makes vulgar comments about Martin's mother and, in particular, his sister, a medical student whom he has never met. ("I'm going to bang the shit out of her and spit on her and treat her like shit" is one of his milder offerings.)

Like a lot of dudes who traffic in this sort of casual misogyny, Incognito and his pals also spout a lot of homophobic trash talk. In addition to hurling racist slurs at a Japanese assistant trainer, Incognito makes it a point to ask him for "rubby rubby sucky sucky." He nicknames another submissive teammate "Loose Booty," and routinely grabs him and asks him for a hug. The homophobia has an anxious, compensatory feel to it. At one point, Pouncey restrains "Loose Booty" and tells Jerry to "come get some pussy." Jerry then touches the victim's ass in a way that simulates anal penetration. Because, you know, that's how you prove you're definitely *not* gay.

What's most striking about *The Wells Report* is its depiction of the volatile friendship between Incognito and Martin.

Teammates describe the two as inseparable. In the course of their stormy fourteen-month relationship, they exchange 13,000 text messages, or nearly 30 a day. They seek each other out "at all hours of the day or night" and discuss "the intimate details of their sex lives, often in graphic terms."

Martin tells the investigators he befriended his tormentor hoping to stem his abuse, as victims often do. He appears genuinely perplexed by Incognito's mood swings. "At one point he pulled his shirt off & tried to beat my ass yesterday," he writes in one text. "Then 5 min later it was like nothing even happened and we went to the strip club." He refers to Incognito as "bipolar."

But the deeper one reads into the report, the more it seems to describe a psychic crisis. Richie Incognito is guilty of bullying. But his true crime seems to be that he harbors forbidden desires for Jonathan Martin.

As he admits to investigators, his term of preference for Martin is "my bitch." When Martin declines his offers to socialize, or to take trips together, Incognito reacts like a spurned lover. His invective reflects a familiar preoccupation. At one point, Incognito pressures Martin to vacation with him in Las Vegas. Here's the exchange of texts that causes Martin to back out:

INCOGNITO: No dude hookers [*male prostitutes*] u faggot
INCOGNITO: Don't blame ur gay tendancies on [*Player A*]
MARTIN: I'm gonna get more bitches in 2 nights than all of you combined

INCOGNITO: Stop it. By bitches u mean cocks in ur mouth
INCOGNITO: U fucking mulatto liberal bitch
INCOGNITO: I'm going to shit in ur eye
INCOGNITO: Goodnight slut

But beneath this profane banter, a genuine tenderness emerges. "Let's get weird tonight," Incognito writes to Martin, at one point. And a bit later, "What's up pussy? I love u." Even after Martin has left the team amid controversy, the two continue to text.

"I miss us," Incognito writes.

As I pored through *The Wells Report*, I kept thinking about this book I reviewed a few years ago called *The Game: Penetrating the Secret Society of Pickup Artists*. The author, Neil Strauss, and his fellow pickup artists obsess over their masculinity and delight in detailing their conquests. But a familiar suspicion lurks beneath the braggadocio. "I was in the game to have more women in my life, not men," Strauss writes. "And though the community was all about women, it was also completely devoid of them ... The point was women; the result was men."

This, it seems to me, is an apt description of the life many pro athletes lead. They have engineered lives in which they work and eat and bathe with other men and live by a set of masculine codes that discourage empathy, introspection, any sign of weakness really. A guy such as Richie Incognito functions like a modern-day Achilles. He may embrace women as sexual objects. But his deepest love is reserved for the men with whom he goes to battle, and it is sometimes difficult for him to regulate the sexual and aggressive drives that roil within him.

As history attests, there are clear social and political ramifications to this internal schism. The reason so many societies have attacked homosexuality is not just because their leaders were sexually insecure (though they were). It's also because the most effective leaders exploited the homoerotic anxieties of their male populations. They defined masculinity as a willingness to do violence without remorse, and offered men the chance to atone for aberrant urges by persecuting homosexuals. This impulse might have found its earliest expression in religious allegories such as Sodom and Gomorrah, but it's not some wild coincidence that fascist cultures and repressive regimes exhibit this same genocidal mania.

Being a jock also provides a safe haven from the emotional and psychological demands of women; it's what an old girlfriend of mine used to call "regression to the mean." Fans experience this as well. The reason I love going out to a bar to watch a football game with Sean (our wives call these excursions "man dates") is precisely because we can just sit there eating onion rings deep-fried in cholesterol, watching the Raiders choke, and *not* discussing anything deeper than the risks of calling a naked bootleg in the red zone. It's a way of clinging to adolescence.

And I can tell you exactly what happens to any dude who dares to speak out about the moral complexities of football. Here's a sampling of the e-mails I received after writing such a piece for *The New York Times Magazine*, printed here verbatim:

> *OMG. I am progressive on social issues but dude—you are the biggest fucking pussy on the face of the earth. Change your tampon you woman.*

> *I read an article you wrote about football and I couldn't help but think of a slutty girl I knew growing up. I thought she had the biggest vagina I'd ever seen before now . . . congrats dude, you have a bigger one.*

> *Why do libs have to ruin everything we do for fun or to take our minds off of the world? I don't even like the Redskins but if that kind of stuff offends the large vagina crowd, I am a fan now.*

Well, then. That was certainly bracing.

I realize that you think I've cherry-picked these. But I swear to you, nearly every piece of hate mail I received made reference to my vagina, which was usually characterized as very large.

As the son of two psychoanalysts, I suppose I am obligated

to speculate on this odd size fixation. Fine. On one level my correspondents simply wish to convey the exaggerated nature of my femininity (i.e., larger vagina = more feminine). Still, it's hard to ignore that a large vagina suggests an unconscious fear of male inadequacy. Is it possible that merely asking these guys to examine their motives for watching football made them feel small?

We can say for sure that these men feel accused. That someone might make them feel guilty for watching football represents the ultimate gender betrayal. The prescribed punishment appears to be the revocation of one's male genitalia.

For the record, my vagina is slightly smaller than average.

If, at its worst, the cult of football preys on male insecurity, prizes physical dominance, and denigrates women, it follows that these tendencies would effect not just how players interact with each other, but with women. And I would be remiss, therefore, in failing to mention the pattern of sexual violence against women perpetrated by football players.

Here's the thing, though: to this point, I've avoided citing criminal complaints. It feels unfair to me to smear the many for the actions of a few. Also, the rate of allegation against players appears exaggerated because of their celebrity. The reason I'm making an exception when it comes to sexual misconduct against women is because of a disturbing pattern that goes far beyond the behavior of individual players: the gross negligence of law enforcement and the public.

The most flagrant recent example involves Jameis Winston, a celebrated quarterback for Florida State University. In December of 2012, a nineteen-year-old undergraduate told Tallahassee police she had been raped after a night of drinking at a popular bar. The young woman claimed her alleged assailant, whom she did not know, transported her to the bedroom of his off-campus apartment, ignored her pleas to stop, held her down, and later carried her to a bathroom where he locked the door and continued the assault. There was physical evidence: bruises indicative of recent trauma, blood on her shorts, and semen on her underwear. A friend of the alleged rapist later told police that he'd taped a portion of the encounter on his phone.

Police never saw this tape, because they barely investigated. Neither did school officials, though federal law requires them to look into any charge of sexual assault against a student. It was the alleged victim who, a month later, called police to identify Winston as the man who raped her, after she saw him on campus.

Her family, fearful she would be antagonized for accusing a football player, asked a lawyer friend to contact the assigned detective, Scott Angulo. According to the family, Angulo—who had done private security work for an FSU booster group—refused to order Winston to submit to DNA testing, because it would generate publicity. He warned that Tallahassee is "a big football town and the victim needs to think long and hard before proceeding against him because she will be raked over the coals and her life will be made miserable." Angulo closed the case without having interviewed Winston or secured his phone records or DNA.

Only after the allegation became public, nine months later, did prosecutors reopen the case. By this time, Winston was one of the best-known football players in the country. Although his DNA matched the DNA found on the alleged victim's clothing, prosecutors did not press charges. FSU did nothing to discipline Winston, though a second woman sought counseling from the school's own victim advocate after a disturbing sexual encounter with him.

In the ensuing months, Winston won the Heisman Trophy and led the Seminoles to a national championship. He has been projected as the number one overall pick in the 2015 NFL draft.

His accuser was publicly reviled—viciously slut-shamed, in some cases—and withdrew from classes. Winston's lawyer accused her of "targeting" his client, though she had no idea he was a football player when she first went to police. She received death threats on social media.

Ladies and gentlemen, I give you the twisted logic of rape culture. The true victim is always the famous baller. And the young woman who goes to the police, bruised and distraught, who submits to a rape exam? She has no right to expect an honest investigation of her allegations. She *deserves* to be verbally abused, ostracized, then discarded. And why?

Because her claims threaten to expose the whole misogynist underpinning of the fan/athlete dynamic, the sickening arrangement by which we give athletes the cultural power to sexually possess women with little fear of the consequences. It's a modern form of tribute; to the victors go the spoils.

Thanks to police incompetence, or worse, we'll never know exactly what happened between Winston and his accuser. FSU has yet to discipline the quarterback, and now joins a host of other colleges under federal investigation for allegedly mishandling sexual assault cases involving athletes. We do know that school officials and students and an entire nation of fans appear more troubled by the prospect of not being able to watch Winston play than by the fact that he might be a rapist.

That's how much we need our football.

Two years ago, in Steubenville, Ohio, a pair of high school football players sexually assaulted a teenage girl incapacitated by alcohol, giddily documented the attack on film, and shared photos on social media. Members of the community rallied around . . . the rapists. They assailed the victim for casting the team and town in a negative light. She was pressured to remain silent and was made an outcast by her peers. Three adults, including the superintendent of schools, were arrested for obstructing the investigation.

Given the preponderance of evidence, the boys were convicted in a juvenile court. Poppy Harlow, a CNN correspondent, described the scene by saying it was "incredibly difficult, even for an outsider like me, to watch what happened as these two young men that had such promising futures, star football players, very good students, literally watched as they believed their lives fell apart."

If the convicts had been drifters or undocumented workers, we can assume they would have been perceived quite differently. But Harlow's little soliloquy reveals a darker possibility: the fact that the assailants *were* star football players might help explain their crimes. The people of Steubenville—fans, parents, coaches—made those boys feel chosen, as if their physical gifts entitled them to special rights, made them impervious to the codes of decency that govern the rest of us, as if their athletic fate mattered more than the dignity of the unconscious teenage girl they raped and humiliated.

7

THE BLIND SPOT

In 1993, a slew of European tourists who had come to Florida on vacation were murdered. The most publicized of these crimes took place in a Miami neighborhood called Liberty City, just a few blocks from a notorious housing project called the James E. Scott Homes, which residents referred to as The Canyon.

I was a reporter for a weekly paper in Miami at the time. I'd reported stories from The Canyon and felt it might behoove the journalistic mission to describe the place in greater detail. I didn't have an angle. I just wanted to hang out long enough—a year of weekly visits, it would turn out—to begin to understand the lives of the women and children who lived there.

Like many public housing projects in poor areas, The Canyon was essentially a village of despondent mothers and restless children. I wound up spending most of my time there with a pack of young boys, none of whom had fathers. To these boys, and their mothers and aunties, one of the few heroic figures was a former NFL player who had returned to run a football program.

He was renowned for one of his rules, which I heard over

and over: he didn't accept any kid older than nine. After that, it was too late. He couldn't undo whatever recalcitrance had been wired or whipped into them. And of course this was terribly sad. Because youth football was viewed as a form of salvation in Liberty City. Pop Warner championships drew thousands of fans. People saw the game as a way to instill discipline and self-respect, to keep wayward boys from taking the wrong path, a golden ticket.

"The only ones ever come back with money is the football players," one mom told me. "Them and the drug dealers."

I keep thinking about it from the point of view of the kids I hung out with, Nookie, Boo Man, the others. These boys lived with mothers or guardians who were too broken to care for them properly. They went to a school that was overcrowded. Their teachers saw them mostly as discipline problems. They had no positive male figures in their lives, no power in the world, no idea how to acquire any.

So I could understand why they were desperate to join a game that gave them a sense of purpose and direction, that earned them the approval and guidance of respected elders who recognized their potential, a game that offered them a chance at riches and fame, however remote. They accepted the need to sacrifice. They had to learn strategy, cooperation, how to channel their aggressive impulses, how to evade or defeat the opponent. They understood that the game in question gave people tremendous pleasure, but that it wasn't economically productive for the local community. And though they preferred not to think about this part, they knew it came with considerable risks to their health.

Despite all this, some of them still wanted to sell crack cocaine.

Am I now suggesting that football is as bad for the African-American community as crack cocaine?

No.

I'm just making the point that neither is a realistic solution to the crises that poor African-American boys face growing up in this country. In fact, they are distractions from the systemic inequalities that keep such boys locked in a cycle of poverty and incarceration.

Without a doubt, football *is* great at getting boys motivated—mostly to play football. It can give the right sort of kid a leg up. But it's "a way out" only for a handful. Less than 10 percent of the 100,000 high school seniors who play football will make a college squad, and fewer still will receive scholarships; 215 will wind up in the pros. That's 1 out of 500 players. The others—the Nookies and the Boo Mans, the ones we prefer not to think about—need better child care programs and better schools and better job training and better wages.

Whatever laudable lessons football imparted to the children of The Canyon, it reinforced the idea that violence was a source of power and a path to destiny. Here's how the commissioner of the local league explained it to Robert Andrew

Powell, whose book, *We Own This Game*, offers a vivid chronicle of Miami's peewee set: "Football is the most natural for them. Basketball puts limits on their aggression; baseball puts limits on their aggression. In football they had better well be aggressive. And with the background of these kids, where these kids come from, aggression comes naturally."

Carlos Guy, the uncle of one player, put it like this: "Somebody a long time ago came to the idea that this— football—was the very best way to show that we could make it out, that we could rise above the slave mentality, segregation, and really be what we want to be. It's not a part of the culture now. It *is* the culture."

I keep trying to imagine what Dr. Martin Luther King would have to say about these statements. His image was all over The Canyon, staring out from the chipped murals that were painted every few years, in anticipation of some visit from a politician. Often, these murals included quotes.

Returning violence for violence multiplies violence, adding deeper darkness to a night already devoid of stars.

Man must evolve for all human conflict a method which rejects revenge, aggression and retaliation.

Nonviolence is a powerful and just weapon . . . It is a sword that heals.

You know, sissy shit like that.

I suspect King would have been heartbroken at the notion that football is the dominant form of empowerment in communities like The Canyon. He might well have viewed the mindset as a form of self-colonization.

The ultimate message football sends to young boys, of whatever color or socioeconomic status, is that they are valuable not for the content of their character, not for their intelligence or creativity, but for how fast they can run and how well they can throw and catch and, especially, how hard they can hit. That's what scouts and recruiters want. That's how you get rescued.

Consider *The Blind Side* by Michael Lewis, a 2006 bestseller that later became a blockbuster film. Lewis tells the story of Michael Oher, a painfully shy African-American teen from the projects of West Memphis who happens to be six feet six inches tall and 345 pounds. Thanks to his unusual combination of size and speed, he is accepted at a private evangelical high school, adopted by a rich white family on the east side of town, and molded into an All-American.

There's an undeniable buzz in tracking Oher's rise from a destitute kid with no prospects to a prodigy besieged by college recruiters. But Lewis never seems to acknowledge that he's telling a different story as well, one of racial exploitation. In fact, he highlights all the rule bending done to keep Oher college-eligible. The administration at his high school accepts him, though he can barely read. When his GPA proves too low for the NCAA, his adoptive father, a canny former college basketball star named Sean Tuohy, finds a loophole. He has Oher tested to prove he's learning disabled, then has him take numerous easy, on-line courses. Lewis treats these measures as ingenious. We are meant to cheer the fact that Oher has gamed the educational process.

Tuohy's indomitable wife also plays a key role in the re-education of Oher:

> Leigh Anne was now making it her personal responsibility to introduce him to the most basic facts of life, the sort of thing any normal person would have learned by osmosis. "Every day I try to make sure he knows something he doesn't know," she said. "If you ask him, *Where should I shop for a girl to impress her?* he'll tell you, *Tiffany's.* I'll go through the whole golf game. He can tell you what six under is, and what's a birdie and what's par."

Leigh Anne treats her adopted son more like a giant kachina doll than a human being.

Oher himself recognizes the ulterior motives swirling around him. "He didn't go so far as to treat Leigh Anne with suspicion but, as Leigh Anne put it, 'With me and Sean I can see him thinking, *If they found me lying in a gutter and I was going to be flipping burgers at McDonald's, would they really have had an interest in me?*' "

No one ever answers this question.

Instead, the Touhys convince Oher to attend their alma mater, Ole Miss, where he becomes a star bound for the NFL. We are meant to view all this as an inspiring underdog saga, spiced with the proper pieties about Christian charity, the power of hope, and individual destiny.

Michael Lewis is one of our finest journalists. He gets that Michael Oher is part of a larger system. "What the NFL prized," he writes, "America's high schools supplied, and America's colleges processed." He understands that assets like Oher have to "go through the tedious charade of pretending to be ordinary college students" to make the pros.

For this reason, I kept wondering why Lewis never addressed that haunting question: why did the Touhys rescue Michael Oher? His avoidance could be due to the fact that he and Sean Touhy are old friends. But I suspect it's deeper than that.

It has to do with a much more fundamental blind spot that prevails when it comes to sports and race in America. And while I could talk here about other sports, such as basketball, football is the prime example, not just because two-thirds of its players are African-American but because it fuels our most insidious and intractable stereotypes about such men: that they are inherently animalistic.

Like most fans, myself included, Lewis prefers not to parse the perverse arrangement by which watching young

African-Americans in tight pants engage in mock combat has become our most profitable form of entertainment. Nobody wants to look at this stuff. Nobody wants to ask the awkward questions.

Such as: What is the relationship between our nation's racial history and our lust for football? What does it mean that football fever tends to run so hot in those states where slavery was legal and Jim Crow died hardest? What does it mean that millions of white fans cheer wildly for African-American men in the context of a football game when, if they encountered these same men on a darkened street, they might very well reach nervously for their cell phone? Is football a way of containing African-American rage? Is this why any African-American athlete who speaks too brashly or associates with friends from the old neighborhood has "character issues"? Does it relieve the racial guilt of white Americans to lavish so much money and adulation on a few African-American men? Is it an oblique form of financial restitution?

And what does it mean that we give so much scrutiny to their bodies? That we think nothing of calling them "studs" and "beasts" and "specimens"? Are we turning them into fetish objects? And what does *that* mean? Can anyone really watch the NFL Combine—in which young, mostly African-American men are made to run and jump and lift weights for the benefit of mostly old white coaches, and us couch potatoes—and *not* see visual echoes of the slave auction?

For that matter: Isn't the whole system by which young African-Americans are harvested from this country's impoverished precincts, segregated from the general population, and exploited for their extraordinarily profitable physical labors, a kind of extravagantly monetized plantation?

Yes, football attracts fans of all races and classes. Yes, players choose to compete and are well paid. But the power dynamics remain eerily familiar: a wealthy white "owner" presides over a group of African-American laborers. Is the "slave mentality" something that a signing bonus erases? Do the millions absolve everyone involved? Does it matter that players risk grievous injury? That they are cast off like beasts of burden?

Does football provide white Americans a continued sense of dominion over African-American men? Do their huge salaries give us the right to pass judgment on them incessantly? To call up radio programs and yell about how they're lazy or money-hungry or thuggish? Do we secretly believe they belong to us? Why do we enjoy seeing them play through pain? Why do we berate them for cowardice when we ourselves wouldn't last ten seconds in an actual game? Is this cycle of hero worship and vilification one way in which white men express anxiety over their perceived physical inadequacies relative to men of color? Is that why the sportscaster Jimmy "The Greek" Snyder got fired, in 1988, for saying "the black is a better athlete ... because he's been bred to be that way" by the slave owner? Was he made a scapegoat for expressing sentiments the rest of us prefer to hide?

Why do white fans react with such shock and horror when African-American players, who are rewarded for ruthless aggression on the field, exhibit these traits elsewhere? Is the obsessive coverage of their violent crimes a public justification for our private prejudices?

What does it mean that 95 percent of our most famous African-American citizens are athletes? Or that, when we see a physically imposing African-American in the lobby of a fancy hotel, or a television studio, we immediately think: *football player*. Why don't we think *doctor* or *software engineer*? Are these assumptions a form of bigotry? If not, why not?

I'm going to get hammered for asking these questions. Fine. Hammer away. But don't pretend that's the same as answering.

Or consider poor Jonathan Martin, last spotted dancing his tortured interracial tango with Richie Incognito. The saddest—and most overlooked—story told by *The Wells Report* is that of his racial reckoning.

Martin grew up in a family that prized education and professional achievement. Had Martin chosen to attend Harvard, where he was accepted, he would have been the university's first fourth-generation African-American student. Instead, he went to Stanford, where he majored in Classics and became a football star widely respected by his comrades.

His problems began when he joined the NFL. African-American teammates accused him of not acting "black enough." He was too intellectual and sensitive. Like that famous punk Martin Luther King, he avoided violent confrontations, which is why Incognito, playing to type, targeted him. Martin blamed his problems on "white private school conditioning, turning the other cheek."

Other players urged Martin to confront Incognito. Instead, he turned his hatred inward, grew disconsolate, and harbored suicidal thoughts. The episode that led him to leave the Dolphins is revealing. Martin was in line at the cafeteria. Incognito was sitting at a table with the other offensive linemen, most of them African-American. He called out to Martin that he didn't want his "stinky Pakistani ass" to join the group. When Martin approached the table anyway, the other linemen rose in unison and, at Incognito's instigation, moved to another table. Martin had been denied a place at the table.

Soon after, media reports noted Incognito's use of racial epithets. *The Wells Report* included two text message exchanges between Incognito and a white teammate in which they joke about murdering black people.

PLAYER B: That's a solid optic made specifically for a .308 battle rifle
INCOGNITO: Perfect for shooting black people
PLAYER B: Lol

And yet African-American teammates still voiced support for Incognito and disdain for Martin. Better a racist than a race traitor. That's what Jonathan Martin was, after all, in the eyes of his comrades. African-American football players don't come from educated families. They don't have a life of the mind. They don't practice nonviolence. With internal standards like that, who needs racial oppressors?

8

THEIR SONS GROW
SUICIDALLY BEAUTIFUL

To this point, I've focused pretty narrowly on the NFL. I've done so because, as Lewis notes above, the pro game drives the whole machine. Its incandescent lure induces a lot of kids to endure a lot of hardship. But there are plenty who play football purely for kicks, who harbor no hope of competing in college or beyond. And it's pretty hard to argue with a kid who simply loves the game. If my son wants to head out to a park for a five-on-five, I'm not about to stop him. I'd rather they play two-hand touch, but if they mix in a few tackles, well, I received my fair share of injuries doing the same.

What bums me out about football at the amateur level is that it's gotten way too organized and cutthroat and just generally corrupted by parasitic adults. And that begins with the fact that the sport has become a part of the educational system of this country, which, I'm sorry, is pathological.

The primary mission of high school and college, I hope we can agree, is to educate students, to stimulate and expand their minds, to prepare them for jobs and lives that contribute to society. (Or at least hold the apocalypse at bay for a few more sunny decades.) But all across the country, particularly in the South, schools have become football factories.

The insane commercialization of the pro game has trickled down through college to high school and led to an athletic arms race. National networks such as ESPN now air high school games. Elite "programs" spend hundreds of thousands on facilities and coaches and recruit from across state lines. The players, in turn, work out year-round. They're as big and strong and fast as the pros of twenty years ago. This has led to a booming industry of scouts, trainers, promoters, and (lest we forget) steroid dealers, whose job is to groom these teens for college stardom. Sixth-period PE, meet late-model capitalism.

Given all this, you might expect enhanced safety standards, if for no other reason than to protect those valuable two-legged commodities. But the nearly 1.1 million boys who play high school football—more than any other sport—are getting hurt more and more often.

The most definitive epidemiological studies suggest that upward of 65,000 concussions are reported per year, though thousands more go undiagnosed because schools lack the medical staff required to recognize the symptoms. Rates have doubled in the past fifteen years. According to a 2013 study funded by the NFL, high school players are nearly twice as likely to incur a concussion as their college counterparts.

Why? Because the NCAA has rules regarding maximum playing and practice times—twenty hours per week during the season; eight hours in the off-season. Although these limits are routinely flouted, they provide some measure of moderation. By contrast, there's no national body to regulate the sport at the high school level.

What's more, the incentives are all wrong. Coaches are under intense pressure to win. They're working with kids who've been taught for years that enduring pain is what makes them worthy, an especially dangerous credo when you cannot conceive of your own mortality. These young men hunger to compete, and a lot of people depend on them to do so: parents, coaches, teammates. The result is that players devote much of their high school careers to preparing for a dozen games each fall. The driving ambition is not education. It's entertainment.

Here's the scariest part: not only do high school players receive more blows to the head than college players, they are more vulnerable to these blows because their brains are still developing.

Three years ago, researchers at Purdue University began monitoring every hit sustained by two local high school teams. The goal was to study the effect of concussions. But when researchers administered cognitive tests to players who had never been concussed, hoping to set up a control group, they discovered that these teens showed diminished brain function as well. As the season wore on, their cognitive abilities plummeted. In some cases, brain activity in the frontal lobes—the region responsible for reasoning—nearly disappeared by season's end. "You have the classic stereotype of the dumb jock and I think the real issue is that's not how they start out," explained Thomas Talavage, one of the professors running the study. "We actually create that individual."

Let's take a deep breath and consider how psychotic that is.

What would happen if some invisible gas leak in the school cafeteria caused diminished brain activity in students? Can we safely assume district officials would evacuate the school until further notice? That parents would be up in arms? That media and lawyers would descend in droves to collect statements from the innocent victims? Can we assume that the community would not gather together en masse on Friday nights to eat hot dogs and watch the gas leak?

So why do Americans not only accept high school football, but, in certain regions, worship it? What is it in our national psychology that gets off on seeing boys engage in such a savage game? I think there's some kind of shame mixed up in it all, the shame of men whose dreams have collapsed.

Here's what James Wright had to say on the subject, in his poem "Autumn Begins in Martins Ferry, Ohio," which I have been unable to get out of my head:

All the proud fathers are ashamed to go home.
Their women cluck like starved pullets,
Dying for love.
Therefore,

Their sons grow suicidally beautiful
At the beginning of October,
And gallop terribly against each other's bodies.

Too heavy? Fine. Let's consider the allure of a show such as *Friday Night Lights*, which revolves around the high school football team in itty bitty Dillon, Texas. I'm not a fan of *FNL*, but I've seen enough episodes to recognize why so many of my friends are. It's well written and acted and it portrays rural America in that seductive way Hollywood so often does: forlorn, earthy, mysteriously rife with gorgeous folks engaged in soap-operatic intrigue.

Also, the producers were canny enough to confront the dark side of high school football right from the start. The pilot features pushy boosters, unctuous recruiters, even a star quarterback who gets paralyzed in the season opener.

To someone who did not grow up in this country, this might not seem like a promising launch. But Americans recognized it as a familiar enticement: a drama whose presentation of "real issues" is actually a form of moral flattery. People who would never allow their own kids to play football watch *FNL* and feel ennobled. Sure, the franchise is built on a slavish devotion to a game that uses and even disables children—but at least they cop to it, man!

FNL also came along in an era when the big concern was traumatic injuries, which could be dismissed as freak accidents. There's no consideration of cognitive impairment on the show. In fact, you barely ever see a student in class. Dillon High exists as a substrate for its football team.

And football isn't just football. It's the local brand of redemption. The pilot includes a scene in which revered quarterback Jason Street gives a bunch of Pop Warner players an inspirational speech, then asks everyone to kneel in prayer. "Do you think God loves football?" one of the moppets asks.

"I think everybody loves football," the QB says.

We are left to consider (or not consider) the theological implications of Street's subsequent spinal cord injury. God's favorite sport apparently mandates that a few of His children be sacrificed.

The star of the show is head coach Eric Taylor, who exudes a beleaguered dignity, which masks the fact that his techniques are actually kind of horrifying. When his hunky star fullback shows up to practice half drunk, Taylor knows just what to do: he has his players circle around the boy and take turns smashing him into the turf, as rock music blares in the background and the coach yells "Get up, son" in his best John Wayne twang. But don't worry. Punishing this kid by turning him into a human tackling dummy doesn't hemorrhage his brain or rupture his spine. It saves his soul. Tough love. Rehab in shoulder pads.

Of note: Buzz Bissinger, author of the book *Friday Night Lights*, upon which the series is loosely based, now believes football should be banned in high school and college. The current system, he says, turns kids into "football animals . . . who have no other purpose in life."

And then I think too about my old pal Pat Flood. We must have watched 10,000 mindless happy hours of sports in our twenties. Now we're suburban dads with all the standard complaints.

I've known Pat's first-born, Jack, since he was a baby. The last time I saw him, a year ago, he stood six feet four inches tall and weighed 275 pounds and I had that invasive thought so peculiar to aging men: *Hey, I used to be able to kick your ass.*

Actually, I suspect Jack weighs more than 275 by now, because he recently received a scholarship to play offensive lineman at a Division I school and is probably under orders to bulk up.

I was surprised to hear that Jack had become such an accomplished player, and curious whether Pat worried about his son's health. Which was stupid. And condescending. Because of course he did. He knows football is, as he put it in a recent e-mail, "brutal and unforgiving." He knows it can cause brain damage. And when he thinks about that risk—really faces it—he knows it isn't worth it.

But this is where things get tricky, because how many of us really live that way? We don't want to believe our children could get hurt, so we don't face it. "Willful denial," Pat calls it. And because Jack attended a private high school known for its football program, Pat became part of a larger community of parents and coaches and boosters who also chose not to think about those risks—even as numerous kids suffered injuries.

When Pat looks at his son, he sees a kid striving for excellence, a kid whose passion has been awakened, who's become a leader, an indifferent student who got up all summer for 6 a.m. practices. A kid so dedicated to his team that he sobbed openly when they lost their final home game.

At Pat's urging, I watched Jack's highlight reel. He was the kind of player who seemed to relish pancaking smaller kids, which was disturbing. But he was also clearly very good. And there was something undeniably thrilling in watching him and his teammates execute complex plays.

I happen to think that Pat is out of his mind and that his son's devotion to football is not only a peril to his health, but may keep him from developing in other important ways. But if my son found that sort of greatness within himself I suspect I'd find a way to support him, too.

This is precisely why those concerned about high school football are pursuing a legal strategy. "You simply can't explain to a child that there is this weird thing called CTE, and in twenty years you might suffer substantial cognitive deficits," says Ivan Hannel, an attorney who authored the paper "CTE: The Developing Legal Case Against High School Football."

Last year, a Mississippi father filed a class action against the National Federation of State High School Associations and the NCAA, in the hopes of forcing both organizations to provide players updated information on health risks and to establish concussion management plans that include insurance coverage for uninsured players.

Hannel says there are considerable challenges. "But you can't have government behind the injury of children in a way that may defeat the purpose of education itself, which is to become more intelligent, not less." He speculates that football at the high school level will eventually migrate to private leagues. This is, in fact, the way sports operate in many European countries.

Now comes the part where I address college football, which means a whole new nation of fans can now despise me.

Yippee!

College football is the arranged marriage of two entities: an institution of higher learning and an athletic industry. It is corrupt and illogical and wildly entertaining and lucrative, which means a legion of lawyers and ad men and sports journalists are handsomely paid to defend and promote its corruption and illogic while the rest of us watch. The beauty of the scheme, from the standpoint of a business student or a sociopath, is that the players themselves get paid nothing.

Actually, that's not true. As we are endlessly reminded by the various Quislings in the employ of the NCAA, they receive *scholarships*. These "student-athletes" are given a chance to succeed in the game of life! Yes, in between the 40–60 hours a week they spend practicing and recovering from practice and working out and attending team meetings and studying the playbook—never mind travel, media duties, and games—you can just imagine how much time and energy they have to devote to course work! After all, what matters most at Auburn is not that their star running back is primed and ready for a nationally televised Bowl game, but that he's primed and ready for that pop quiz in Anthropology. You can imagine how concerned all his coaches must be about his academic progress, given that their own career trajectories depend entirely on climbing the national football rankings.

Fun fact: up to a third of Division I football players never graduate.

I don't mean to be flippant. I'm sure there are many college players who pursue their studies strenuously. My point is that the system doesn't require them to. The notion that they've enrolled in college to learn more about the world of ideas is a fraud we all consent to so we can watch them compete on Saturday.

And it's a fraud that degrades the essential educational mission. It suggests that what really matters, what makes a college worth attending and supporting, isn't scholarship or research or intellectual transmission, but athletics. Which is why, when you hear the name of a large state school such as the University of Texas or Florida or Michigan you don't think of a college at all. You think of a football team.

To return to the issue of free labor, let us consider the recent claim, made by football players at Northwestern, that they be considered employees of the university, and thus allowed to unionize. This is not, as the media has reported it, a "controversy." The players recruited by Northwestern work over forty hours per week, even in the off-season. In any other context, we would call that a job.

The NCAA is desperate to fight this case, because it would crush the fragile foundational myth of the "student-athlete." It would make college football seem too much like what it actually is: one of the nation's fastest-growing industries. The top ten programs alone increased their revenues (self-reported, naturally) from $290 million to nearly $800 million in the ten years from 2001 to 2011. That's more than 150 percent growth.

In 2012, ESPN paid $7.3 billion to broadcast the newly implemented college football playoffs for the next twelve years. Major conferences such as the SEC and Big Ten have launched their own hugely profitable networks. I would estimate the eventual total revenues for the nation's 125 major programs (TV rights, ticket sales, merchandise, video game licensing) at a gazillion dollars.

Boosters point to all this moolah as a justification for the programs. *Look here*, they say. *Our football team is keeping this institution afloat.* The truth is that it's tremendously expensive to run a football program, what with multimillion dollar coaching contracts and recruiting visits and so on. The Stanford program, for instance, generated $25 million in 2011–2012, and spent $18 million. Ohio State spent $34 million. Alabama spent $37 million. *In one year.*

To be sure, the biggest programs do turn a profit. But that profit doesn't provide financial aid for underprivileged philosophy students, or new labs for the chemistry department. It goes mainly to other athletics. More significantly, as economists Rodney Fort and Jason Winfree have noted, only a small share of the nation's college football programs turn a profit at all. And most of it goes right back into the business.

Andrew Zimbalist, a leading sports economist at Smith College, notes that spending per student at schools with major programs stands at roughly $14,000 per year. The figure is over $90,000 for student athletes. In the country's most famous conference, the SEC, schools spend nearly twelve times as much on athletes as they do on students who came to study, say, engineering or epidemiology. Colleges with big football programs also spend hundreds of millions on big stadiums—subsidized by (wait for it) taxpayers and even other students in the form of student fees.

This is a point the writer Malcolm Gladwell makes, that virtually nobody else seems to care about: every college in America is supported by taxpayer dollars, and granted tax-exempt status. We do this because we value the collegiate mission, which is not to have a number one football team, but to graduate students who will go about the dull business of contributing to our society.

So who really benefits economically from college football?

The NFL.

Not only is it an ideal developmental league, it's a humungous free publicity machine. The college game turns players such as Andrew Luck and Robert Griffin, Jr. and Johnny Manziel into brand names before they ever set foot on a pro field. Much of the reason the NFL dominates the sporting landscape is because its minor league system is, itself, the third most popular sport in America, and will probably overtake baseball before long.

Of course, when we think about the big money and glamour of the college game, we're really thinking about the elite teams. What fans rarely see, and almost never think about, is how the game operates in the hundreds of smaller programs where players run even greater risks with no chance of going pro.

In August of 2011, the football coaches at Frostburg State, in western Maryland, held a series of two-a-day practices intended to whip the team into fighting trim. You may be forgiven for not having heard of the Frostburg Bobcats. They are one of the nation's 239 Division III teams.

The most infamous of the drills was reserved for fullbacks. One fullback pretended to be a linebacker. This meant he had to stand defenseless while another fullback leveled him. According to a lawsuit filed by the family of a fullback named Derek Sheely, here's what happened:

On the first day, running backs coach Jamie Schumacher ordered players to hit "hat first," meaning they should lead with their helmets. The drill was not over until each player had engaged in thirty to forty collisions. On the second day, one such collision opened a gash on Sheely's forehead, which bled profusely. Sheely had suffered a concussion the previous season, but the trainer bandaged him up and sent him back onto the practice field—without administering a concussion test. The same thing happened twice more on day three, and again on day four. At one point, Sheely told his coach he had a headache and didn't feel right. "Stop your bitching and moaning and quit acting like a pussy and get back out there Sheely," Shumacher said.

Sheely did. A few minutes later, he collapsed and never regained consciousness. Like the young female rugby player whose brain Ann McKee autopsied, Sheely appeared to have died from second-impact syndrome, a sudden swelling of the brain caused by receiving a concussion before recovering from a previous one.

Sheely's family filed a wrongful death suit against the NCAA, which submitted a thirty-page brief in response. According to this document, which might be described, charitably, as consistency-challenged, the NCAA "denies that it has a legal duty to protect student-athletes" and yet goes on to concede, on the very same page, that it was "founded to protect young people from the dangerous and exploitative athletic practices of the time." The brief is a clumsy attempt to shift liability from the organization to individual schools.

In fact, the NCAA's response to the issue of brain trauma manages to make the NFL look virtuous. In 2010, the governing body did mandate that its member schools adopt concussion-management plans, and set out certain rules. For instance, concussed athletes were barred from returning to action for, well, the rest of the day anyway.

But it turns out that the NCAA doesn't actually enforce these plans, or even oversee them. Its director of health and safety, David Klossner, admitted as much in a deposition last year. Asked point-blank whether the NCAA had ever disciplined any of its member schools regarding these concussion plans, or even considered doing so, Klossner answered, "Not to my knowledge."

It might be worth mentioning at this point that the NCAA faces a score of federal lawsuits stemming from concerns about concussion care. The reason we know about Klossner's testimony is because hundreds of pages of internal NCAA documents were made public last year, as part of an effort to convert a concussion lawsuit into a class action. E-mails reveal that other senior NCAA staffers actually mocked Klossner's safety efforts.

I am (of course) a total effing hypocrite when it comes to college football, because over the past five years I've become increasingly sucked in by the Stanford team, which is not my alma mater but where, as you'll recall, I sold hot dogs and watched John Elway gallivant so many years ago. The reason I got interested in the team was pathetically predictable: they got very good.

Last year, I decided to stop watching them. I kept see-ing players get concussed during games, which I find more disturbing at the college level because I've actually taught undergraduates. It also dawned on me that the Stanford ad-ministration had made the disheartening decision to build an elite football program apparently because being an aca-demically revered university wasn't cutting it with the folks in corporate branding.

Then again, I've never felt an insane devotion to the col-lege game, like my friend Sean, whose overweening love of the Virginia Tech Hokies caused that broken hand I men-tioned earlier.

An even more curious case is Evan, a respected endocri-nologist who runs a medical research lab at Harvard. I think of Evan as the kind of guy who does not suffer fools, or fool-ishness. And yet he has, over the years, been so infatuated with Michigan football as to haunt the message boards that serve as grievance depots for the truly afflicted. He told me he first got hooked his second year of medical school at Mich-igan. "Everything else basically sucked but at least there was this event, once a week, that everyone cared about. It was like you were instantly part of this huge tribe. I got wrapped up in it very quickly."

Sure, I said, but you were studying to become a *doctor*.

"Yeah," Evan said, unconvincingly. "There was this part of me that realized that players were getting hurt, and ripped off, and that football wasn't the proper purview of a world-class university. But there was this other part of me that just felt unmitigated glee when they won. And those two parts of me are often not talking to each other."

Evan said his passion for Michigan had started to ebb—until his son became a fan. Three years ago, they took a trip out to Ann Arbor to see the Wolverines beat Ohio State, an experience both of them look upon as a kind of holy pilgrimage. Why begrudge them this? After all, I still bond with my dad over sports. It's a language to which we can always safely return. But it's also true that I now often wish we had found more personal ways to connect, ways that didn't do such harm to our principles.

9

ALL GAMES ASPIRE TO A CONDITION OF WAR

As a rule, my brothers and I avoided playing sports against each other. There was just too much pent-up feeling between us. But for whatever reason, when I was about fourteen, we took part in a pickup football game with a bunch of our friends.

At some point, my team kicked off and my twin brother Mike wound up with the ball. He'd been a chubby, uncoordinated kid, indifferent to sports. But over the previous year he had grown into his body and assumed a strength and coordination that caught Dave and me off guard. On this play in particular, it was as if a slumbering giant had been roused. He didn't fake anybody out, just ploughed through two tacklers, Earl Campbell style, and shrugged off a third like a flimsy cape. Then he was in the open field with only one man left.

He ran straight at me along the grass with his top lip tucked. There was no effort at evasion. And I myself was frozen with panic, in a kind of shock I guess. I was the designated jock of the family, but he outweighed me by thirty pounds and kept barreling toward me, and as I remember it—by which I mean, as I have constructed the memory—everyone else was just waiting for me to get pancaked.

Then Mike was on the ground, shaking his head a little, and I was standing over him as murmurs of wonder rose from the other kids.

Here's what had happened: just as Mike reached me, I took a half step to my right and my left arm found the crook of his neck so that, as his lower body raced ahead, he was violently upended. The maneuver is known as a clothesline tackle. It was not expressly forbidden in our game (because nothing is *expressly* forbidden in pickup games) but it was understood that even in a tackle game you didn't aim for heads or necks.

Mike and I had been so close as kids that we'd walked to kindergarten with our shoulders pressed together. We'd loved each other, and then that love had become too dangerous and was warped into a competitive rage so deeply ingrained as to seem a way of being.

For years, I had taken a romantic view of this play. It was a gesture toward intimacy, a kind of veiled embrace. But that's not what it was at all. My brother had charged at me and I had taken him down with a vengeance that stunned both of us. To this day, I have no memory of the tackle itself because my mind went perfectly blank, which is what happens to an athlete in the vital moment of contact: you abandon the distractions of thought, of moral calculation.

It is the moment when a human becomes a weapon, the moment when a civilian becomes a soldier.

NFL players themselves know this. They call themselves soldiers all the time. They talk about being in the trenches, going to war, all that martial jargon. They know that all the fancy strategy eventually gives way to the essential question: Which side hits hardest?

Ray Lewis puts it like this: "The long runs, the touchdowns and all that, that's the glamour. But the game is about taking a man down, physically and mentally." Michael Strahan is even more candid. "It's the most perfect feeling in the world to know you've hit a guy just right, that you've maximized the physical pain he can feel ... You feel the life just go out of him." Aggression isn't just some unfortunate-but-necessary aspect of football. What Strahan is describing is the definition of *sadism*, the pleasure one takes in harming another. And he and Lewis aren't hysterical outliers. They are two of the most famous players of all time. Lewis works for ESPN. Strahan just joined the team at *Good Morning America*.

The rise of football in this country isn't just about entertainment or money. It's a modern expression of what historian Richard Slotkin termed "regeneration through violence." Slotkin's interest was in the way British colonists crafted a mythology that reflected their desire for autonomy and territorial expansion in a strange and untamed landscape. Americans have always defined themselves by means of savage confrontation, from the heroics of the Revolutionary War through the ad hoc battles of the frontier and the mass carnage of the Civil War.

As military conflicts have migrated to foreign countries farther and farther away, and the visceral experience of war has grown more abstracted, football has stepped in to ritualize these forms of combat. It's become the national pastime not just because it suits this age (frantic, competitive, data-saturated) but because it reflects the bloodthirsty id that's always defined American identity.

Those holy moments before the Super Bowl—when a famous soprano sings about the rockets red glare and the Blue Angels perform a flyover and we see visions of our brave boys in blue (or red or white) weeping as they prepare to go to battle—represent a kind of national passion play.

Here's how Paul "Tank" Younger, one of the first African-Americans to compete in the NFL, put it: "My inspirational speech was when they played the national anthem. That really got me fired up. It always fired me up and I wanted to go and hit somebody. Shit, when they sang *o'er the land of the free and the home of the brave*, I'm ready to go knock the hell out of somebody."

Jerry Kramer, one of Vince Lombardi's players, described the execution of the team's signature play, the power sweep, like this: "It's really all of life. We all have to do things together to make this thing we call America great. If we don't, we're fucked."

•   •   •

As Americans, the thing we do together, more and more each year, is *watch* football. Fans tend to be less forthcoming than players about their hunger for violence. But the video feed tells the truth. The reason ferocious hits get broadcast over and over, often in slow motion, is because fans love to see them. Like all rubberneckers, we tell ourselves we're watching out of concern for the injured party. (Who knows, maybe we could recommend a good neurologist?) But the TV people know our appetites.

That's why they have those parabolic microphones stationed on the sidelines, so we can hear the crunch of impact. It's why the *Monday Night Football* intro for years featured helmets ramming into each other and exploding and why the NFL Network airs shows promoting the league's most feared tacklers. It's why ESPN—in the pre-concussion era, anyway—aired a segment called *Jacked Up* that featured grown men (among them Steve Young, a man forced to retire from football owing to multiple concussions) chanting, "You just got . . . *jacked up!*" over clips of players being crushed.

It's why the single most viewed football play of the past few years was not a game-winning touchdown, but a hit delivered by a college lineman named Jadeveon Clowney that was so pulverizing the runner's helmet flew off his head as he himself flew backward. ESPN conducted an instant poll asking viewers if this tackle was "the best ever" and later awarded Clowney an ESPY—the Oscar of the sports world—for Best Play of the Year. In May, Clowney became the number one pick in the NFL draft.

• • •

Social scientists have conducted numerous studies to determine why male subjects enjoy violent hits so much. The reasons are many and overlapping. They represent a symbolic catharsis, a purging of violent emotion. They allow us to experience vicarious feelings of dominance. The physical risks create a higher grade of a drama.

But most fans hate to acknowledge these motives, so the football industry does lots to enable us. To begin with, there's all that equipment to shield us from seeing the worst damage. Even more influential are the sportscasters, whom we perceive as strategic authorities, but who function mostly as damage-control experts. Hits that viewers might regard, objectively, as aggravated assaults are safely reinterpreted as "sanctioned violence" in the context of the game.

Good old Sean (who, if he has gotten this far in the book, already hates me) recently showed me a clip that could serve as a master class in how to normalize gratuitous violence for the viewer.

The play occurs in last year's Sun Bowl, when Virginia Tech's star quarterback, Logan Thomas, throws a screen pass and is—to use the athletic term of convenience—*blown up* by a UCLA linebacker named Jordan Zumwalt. The camera tracks the pass, so you don't see the hit initially. But you hear a gruesome crack, followed by an *Ohhhh* from the sportscasters and the crowd, an involuntary exclamation endemic to football that combines shock, distress, and delight in about equal measures.

"Someone got even with Logan Thomas on that one!" whoops Gary Danielson, the color commentator. This is a reference to an earlier play in which Thomas, running in the open field, leveled a defender. By the code of the game, the shame Thomas visited upon the defense warranted this revenge.

But what emerges from subsequent replays of the hit (there are no fewer than ten in a three-minute span) is that this is rather like equating a demolition derby to a hit-and-run. Thomas, having just thrown the ball, is not braced for impact. He's utterly helpless, doesn't have the ball, and thereby should be off-limits to defenders. Zumwalt doesn't veer away from Thomas or aim for the numbers. He launches the crown of his helmet at Logan's head and winds up striking his faceguard—that's the crack we heard—while his arms and shoulders transfer enough kinetic energy to knock Logan flat. From one angle Logan appears to have been vaporized. The hit scores a perfect ten on the Strahan Scale. Logan lies on the ground for more than two minutes, while medical personnel kneel over him. He appears, at one point, to be writhing in pain.

Danielson is duly troubled by what he's seen. He can't believe that Zumwalt has been flagged for unnecessary roughness. "I mean, what are you supposed to do if you're a linebacker?" he implores.

The true victim here—does this sound familiar?—is the assailant. "I don't know if they're escorting Zumwalt off the field. I hope not, because that was a clean play." A bit later,

Danielson explains why the hit is not only justifiable, but laudable. Logan is "tough to bring down." Defensive players "have to be physical with him."

One hears in Danielson's jargon the expected deployment of euphemism, and in his tone the kind of earnest exculpatory vigor so common among football analysts. He's trying to reassure himself, as well as us fans, that the traumatic brain injury Logan just sustained (and sustains over and over in the replays) is, within the ethical borders of the game, permissible.

At a certain point, we see the hit at an especially grisly angle. Danielson is overcome by the sheer brutality. "Oh my goodness!" he exclaims. Then he collects himself and reverts to the company line. "I don't know what the message is here. The defensive players are going, 'What's the rules? Are we supposed to hit him *softly*?'"

Danielson is careful to remind us that no one *wants* Thomas to get hurt, a statement that is both wishful and false. Wishful because what fans want, actually, is a kind of magic we must leave behind in childhood: collisions so extreme as to seem lethal that inflict no harm. And false, because Zumwalt did to Thomas *precisely* what he wanted to do, what he has been trained his whole life to do. And what his coaches and teammates and every UCLA fan on earth count on him to do. (To say nothing of the gamblers who laid money on UCLA.)

Attrition is a basic strategic goal in football: injuring the other team's stars so badly they cannot compete. This is what distinguishes football from virtually every other major team sport, and brings it closer to war.

For the record, when Thomas left the game, the score was 7–7. Without him, Virginia Tech lost 42–12. After the game, Zumwalt, named co-MVP, had this to say to a national audience: "We played lights out."

We choose to view sportscasters as impartial experts, because affording them this status allows us to cling to the notion of sanctioned violence. We get to consume savagery without feeling we *are* savage. But what the sportscasters actually do is stage-manage our experience of watching football.

In this same way, we turn to sports pundits to provide us psychologically soothing interpretations of the sport's ethical dilemmas. When the problem is brain trauma, for instance, the answer is enhanced safety measures.

For the most part, what pundits do is shift our focus away from the game's inherent venality to a few convenient scapegoats: greedy players rather than a rapacious industry, a deviant individual rather than a culture that fosters criminal hubris, bad apples rather than a diseased orchard.

Pundits reserve the most bile for those players and coaches who expose the true nature of the game. That's what happened to Gregg Williams, the former defensive coordinator of the New Orleans Saints, when it was revealed that he was offering bounty payments to players who injured opponents. "Kill the head, the body will die!" Williams told his players in a rather overheated pre-game speech.

Williams was saying, in more brutish slang, what every defensive coach says. He might still be coaching for the Saints if he hadn't offered his players money, and gotten caught on tape. (As Malcolm Gladwell has noted, the excoriation of Michael Vick for his involvement in dogfighting reeked of the same scapegoat fervor.)

The most chilling moments in football are ones in which the images can't be reframed or rationalized. Last season, for instance, Packers tight end Jermichael Finley collided with George Iloka of the Cincinnati Bengals. Finley rose from the ground and staggered toward the sideline. It was clear he was severely concussed. Even as Finley flopped to the ground, another Bengal player ran past him to greet Iloka in jubilation.

So the question isn't just *why* we dig the violence, but what it means and what it does to us. When we see plays like those described above, we are buying into a value system, making a tacit agreement that winning matters more than someone getting hurt. We consent to this premise over and over again until we no longer really have to consent. The psychic structures within us consent. Football valorizes courage and self-sacrifice. It enforces conformity and desensitizes us to violence. It militarizes the way we think and feel. Here's how George Orwell put it back in 1945:

Serious sport has nothing to do with fair play. It is bound up with hatred, jealousy, boastfulness, disregard of all rules, and sadistic pleasure in violence. In other words, it is war without shooting.

To which we might add Cormac McCarthy's more refined view:

Games of chance require a wager to have meaning at all. Games of sport involve the skill and strength of the opponents and the humiliation of defeat and the pride of victory are in themselves sufficient stake because they inhere in the worth of the principals and define them. But trial of chance or trial of worth all games aspire to the condition of war for here that which is wagered swallows up game, player, all.

This link has been obvious from the earliest days of the game. Teddy Roosevelt, who, as president, rescued football from its own caveman excess, nonetheless believed it prepared men for battle. He took as evidence the fact that many of his fellow Rough Riders had played. "In life, as in a football game, the principle to follow is: Hit the line hard; don't foul and don't shirk, but hit the line hard!"

Football is nowhere near as brutal as, say, boxing. But it is the one sport that most faithfully recreates our childhood fantasies of war as a winnable contest. And its evolution reflects the gradual absorption of military precepts: victory achieved by means of force, incremental seizure of territory, escalating violence, and so on.

The peace movement that arose in response to the Vietnam War put a spotlight on the ideological link between football and our Armed Forces. Ron Powers, the author of a history of television called *Supertube*, described the NFL's primary network, CBS, as "a passive accomplice to another payload of values that refuted most of the social revolution's aims. As seen on TV in the sixties, the National Football League leaped quickly from the status of fringe sport to a full-blown expression of America's corporate and military ethos."

In the seventies, the hero of the Dallas Cowboys, "America's Team," was a Vietnam veteran named Roger Staubach, who became the embodiment of the league's reverence for all things military. The alliance took on a cinematic flamboyance during the Reagan Administration.

A former player, sportscaster, and movie star, Ronald Reagan understood the optics of football as only a trained propagandist could. Without seeming the least bit "political," he used the game to capture the virility and patriotism he wished to project as a leader. He routinely chucked footballs from his presidential podium, took his nickname, "The Gipper," from All-American Notre Dame player George Gipp, whom he portrayed onscreen, and held his second inauguration on Super Bowl Sunday of 1985. (Never one to miss a photo op, Reagan ditched the inaugural ball to perform the coin toss via remote.)

It was Reagan's successor, George H.W. Bush, who

initiated the era of overt collaboration between the NFL and the military. In January of 1991, eleven days before Super Bowl XXV, Bush the Elder ordered an attack on Iraq, initiating what became known as the First Gulf War. League officials, working with network executives and the White House, converted the game into a five-hour "infomercial for war," as one critic put it. In addition to images of soldiers in the desert during the pregame show, President Bush addressed the nation at halftime, describing the war as his Super Bowl.

The Armed Forces, recognizing young football fans as the ideal target demographic for recruits, became a major sponsor of the game, while the League took an official position that "supporting the military is part of the fabric of the NFL."

The terrorist attacks of 2001 saw the advent of what we might call Gridiron Agitprop. In cooperation with the second Bush administration, the NFL and Fox aired a three-hour pregame show called "Heroes, Hope, and Homeland" in 2002. When the Bush administration launched the second invasion of Iraq in 2003, the league held a kickoff concert at the National Mall and honored soldiers with an hourlong special. The NFL helped politicians and generals convince the public that the complex issue of going to war could be as emotionally simple as sending the home team overseas for a big game.

By now, fans have become habituated to the cloying tributes and flyovers and remote feeds from army bases, to the slick montages of soldiers played over NFL theme music, to the inexorable blending of gridiron and military iconography. We think nothing of the fact that a private industry intended to provide entertainment has become a publicity arm of the United States military. Our job is to chant "USA! USA!" at any mention of our brave men and women in uniform.

What the NFL has done, in other words, is to help mainstream war, to make it seem like a rational arrangement that young Americans are killing and being killed overseas in perpetuity.

Football has been a boon for the military. But the military has been a boon for football, too. Over the past dozen years, as Americans have sought a distraction from the moral incoherence of the conflicts in Iraq and Afghanistan, the game itself has served as a loyal and dramatically satisfying proxy.

After all, the wars initiated by the Bush administration—scrubbed of any actual carnage by military censors—wound up looking less like warfare on television than some early-generation Atari game, or shapeless documentary. The disingenuous political justifications for the Iraq war, in particular, and the abject incompetence of both occupations, left many Americans with a kind of unrequited combat zeal. We wanted to cheer for the troops, but could find little authentic reason to. Football provided a morally acceptable and gratifying outlet for these patriotic energies, a clearly defined contest of will, a side to root for and against, a clear result, with no unsightly corpses.

Which is why the recent revelation that football can and does cause brain damage has cast such a long shadow.

The struggle playing out in living rooms across the country is that of a civilian leisure class that has created, for its own entertainment, a caste of warriors too big and strong and fast to play a child's game without grievously injuring one another. The very rules that govern our perceptions of them might well be applied to soldiers: Those who exhibit impulsive savagery on the field are heroes. Those who do so off the field are classified as criminals.

The civilian and the fan participate in the same system. We off-load the mortal burdens of combat, mostly to young men from the underclass, whom we send off to battle with hosannas and largely ignore when they return home disfigured in body or mind.

It is a paradoxical dynamic. After all, part of what it means to be a football fan is that we have a sophisticated appreciation for the game, and a deep respect for the players who compete at the highest level. The most rabid fans recognize, in a way others don't, the miraculous gifts of courage and grace that athletes summon in the face of danger. You would think that such reverence would make us more concerned about the fate of such men.

But it turns out that our adulation for football players (for all athletes, really) is highly conditional. As soon as they no longer excel on the field, they become expendable. It is this same mindset that allows us, as a nation, to go to war under false pretenses and suffer so little distress at the resulting human ruin.

·   ·   ·

No single episode speaks to this culture of collusion more pointedly than the life and death of Pat Tillman, an idealistic NFL star who enlisted in the Army following the terrorist attacks of 2001. The military turned Tillman into a recruiting tool, while the sports media canonized him as a soldier saint who had forsaken a lucrative contract to serve his country. Here at last was a figure who embodied the psychic kinship between football and war. And though few paused to wonder why he was the only player to enlist in the "War on Terror," no one doubted that he had taken manly virtue to the max.

The reality was more muddled. Tillman was an unusually thoughtful athlete in search of a deeper purpose. He had signed up to fight terrorism. Like thousands of other soldiers, he wound up in Iraq instead, where he quickly grew disillusioned. In his private journal, he fretted that he would be "called upon to take part in something I see no clear purpose for . . . I believe we have little or no justification other than our imperial whim." He hated the crass effort to market him as a jock G.I. Joe and confided to a friend that he feared if he were killed the Army would parade his body in the street.

By 2004, Tillman had been redeployed to Afghanistan. That April, he was killed in what military officials described as a firefight near the Pakistan border. He was awarded the Silver Star, a medal reserved for soldiers who exhibit "gallantry in action against an enemy of the United States." ESPN broadcast his memorial service live. His former team, the Arizona Cardinals, erected a Pat Tillman Freedom Plaza outside its stadium. Even in death, Tillman's identity was being carefully constructed. He became a square-jawed alpha martyr to the cause of freedom.

In fact, according to the Army's own subsequent investigation, Tillman had been killed by his own side, shot three times by comrades who, in the bedlam of an ill-advised mission, mistook him for an enemy fighter. The last soldier to see him alive was instructed not to reveal how Tillman had been killed. His uniform and body armor were burned, as was the notebook in which he recorded his thoughts about his tour in Afghanistan. An officer who knew Tillman had been a victim of friendly fire warned President Bush not to mention him. Military officials actually ordered members of his platoon to lie to his family during the memorial, and waited weeks to tell them the truth.

The irony is that Tillman—had he lived, had his journal not been torched—might well have become the most famous critic of the War on Terror. According to his mother, he had arranged a meeting with Noam Chomsky, one of the few public intellectuals to question American militarism and intervention.

Here's how Tillman's father put it:

They blew up their poster boy.

It's easy enough to see the duplicity of the military in these machinations. But suppose Pat Tillman had survived, returned to play in the NFL, and wound up with brain damage at age fifty. Would we fans see him as a victim of friendly fire? Would we acknowledge our role in his demise? Or would we construct our own personal cover-ups?

• • •

And what to make of the strange case of Rashard Mendenhall? NFL fans will remember Mendenhall as a former All-Pro running back for the Pittsburgh Steelers who abruptly left the game at age twenty-six. He, too, passed up on a multimillion dollar contract. But they're not about to erect a Rashard Mendenhall Freedom Plaza outside Heinz Stadium. He's more likely to be written off as a quitter, or a heretic.

Why? Because he refused to follow the code of conduct that governs how a football player, particularly an African-American one, should behave. When the military killed Osama Bin Laden in 2011, Mendenhall was the only player in the league to publicly question the cheering mobs. "What kind of person celebrates death?" he tweeted. "I believe in God. I believe we're ALL his children. And I believe HE is the ONE and ONLY judge."

That same year, Mendenhall again infuriated fans and pundits by voicing support for his fellow running back, Adrian Peterson, who had compared the NFL to "modern-day slavery." Peterson was trying to make a simple point: owners reaped billions of dollars on the backs of their players, yet refused to share financial information with them. He quickly apologized for the comments. But Mendenhall was again, to quote his Internet critics, "uppity."

"[Peterson] is correct in his analogy of this game," he tweeted. "Anyone with knowledge of the slave trade and the NFL could say that these two parallel each other."

Mendenhall played football for seventeen years. He knew the rules: shut up and play the game and collect your dough.

But he knew he was being used, and used up. So he committed the ultimate sin: he deserted.

> *Over my career, because of my interests in dance, art and literature, my very calm demeanor, and my apparent lack of interest in sporting events on my Twitter page, people in the sporting world have sometimes questioned whether or not I love the game of football. I've always been a professional. But I am not an entertainer. I never have been. Playing that role was never easy for me. The box deemed for professional athletes is a very small box. My wings spread a lot further than the acceptable athletic stereotypes and conformity was never a strong point of mine . . . So when they ask me why I want to leave the NFL at the age of 26, I tell them that I've greatly enjoyed my time, but I no longer wish to put my body at risk for the sake of entertainment.*

Another way of putting it would be that he insisted on being judged by the content of his character.

Maybe it makes sense to think of football players as human sacrifices. Maybe that's what we're up to. That would certainly help explain why so many athletes and fans place their faith in Jesus Christ. He was a human sacrifice, too.

For two thousand years, Christians have looked upon the ravaged body of Christ as proof of his devotion to a greater cause. This image was obsessively represented in art (take a look at Rembrandt's *Passion Series*), in religious pageants, and upon the crucifixes that signified the place of worship in the home. Maybe it makes sense to think of television as the new domestic altar, around which we congregate to view images of young men bloodied and broken in service to that highest American cause: victory.

After all, sacrificial rituals don't have to involve throwing virgins into volcanoes or cutting the hearts out of warriors on the tops of temples. They can take subtler forms. Christian polemicists such as Tertullian considered the gladiators of Rome to be human sacrifices. Pagans took a more contemporary view. To them, the crucial difference was between certain death and the risk of death. The thrill of the arena resided in seeing how a man would behave in the face of danger.

Doesn't that sound like football?

Maybe the modern sacrificial impulse is a natural response to the stark Darwinist pressures of capitalism, the arena in which all of us, like it or not, must now compete. Maybe football represents the illusion of order imposed upon our chaotic aggression. Maybe watching games isn't just an evasion but a way of managing our panic about resource depletion, climate change, plague, the looming prospect that the serpent within our souls will doom the human experiment.

This would help explain our obsession with imagined dystopias that feature sacrificial sport, from *Rollerball* to *The Hunger Games*. Maybe this is why we spend more and more of our time consuming sacrificial entertainments, programs in which the central allure is watching people damage each other and themselves.

Cultures don't practice human sacrifice simply out of cruelty, after all. Enacting these rituals creates a powerful bond among the sacrificing community. Maybe football has become the only spiritual adhesive strong enough to unite Americans, a modern temple in which neighbors join together during Sunday services to slake fierce and ancient longings once served by the Church.

Let me be clear about this: I believe our insatiable appetite for football is symptomatic of our imperial decadence, of our quiet desperation for shared dramas in an age of social and psychic atomization, for animal physicality in an era of digital abstraction, for binary thought in an age of moral fragmentation.

But I also believe that watching football indoctrinates Americans, that it actually *causes* us to be more bellicose and tolerant of cruelty, less empathic, less willing and able to engage with the struggles of an examined life.

Let me nominate myself as a prime example. I was opposed to the wars in Afghanistan and Iraq, and troubled by the nationalist wrath that erupted from every cultural portal in the weeks and months after the terrorist attacks of 2001. I wrote a few articles to this effect, and did a lot of grumbling.

What I didn't do was enact my values, protest, pursue my version of social justice, though I had plenty of time to do so.

Instead, I spent countless hours tracking the Oakland Raiders and making my pathetic Sunday pilgrimages to the Good Times Emporium to watch the team's baroque implosions.

Let's compare this to what my father was up to in *his* early thirties. He organized students against the Vietnam War and was arrested for blocking the entrance to a nearby military base, actions that cost him dearly in his academic career. He supported and participated in the back-to-the-land movement. He worked on a book about communal living. And he did all this while working and helping to raise three small sons.

And yet, for all this, it's also true that my dad watched football and other sports, and that his ideals, like the rest of the Republic's, got somewhat sidetracked by the games. His fandom marked the beginning of my own. Those games drew me closer to my dad, but they also led me to see aggression as a form of pride rather than a symptom of grief.

One of the most disturbing memories of my childhood is a vicious brawl I had with my older brother Dave, which took place in our TV room. At some point, my dad came into the room. He didn't break things up. As I remember it, he urged me on. He knew that Dave bullied me a lot and I think he liked seeing me stand up for myself. He was proud of me afterward, but I wept in humiliation. And I'm still struggling with all this shit years later. I still have to fight the impulse to watch clips of the Raiders' glory days on YouTube—or worse, old boxing matches.

But sometimes I look around at the prevailing landscape

and I think: we're all hopped up on the same bad brew of rage and fear and grievance. We're ready to shoot each other in traffic. We're treating the provision of health care to poor people as some kind of conspiracy. We've forgotten that we once fought a War on Poverty. Maybe D.H. Lawrence was right. Maybe the essential American soul is "hard, isolate, stoic, and a killer."

And then there are other times, when I remember the symptoms associated with CTE—loss of memory, problems focusing, mood swings, impaired judgment—and lean toward a slightly more hopeful conclusion.

Maybe our entire Republic is concussed.

10

BILL SIMMONS DRAWS THE LINE

I have no right to tell anyone what to do, especially when it comes to football. I've supported the game for four decades. No overnight conversion is going to undo that. But I do have a right, like all Americans, to speak about what I see.

Still, it's worth asking why I've written this manifesto now, as opposed to, say, a decade ago when it would have been genuinely subversive. I've wondered the same thing myself.

Partly it's because, though I enjoy watching the game more than ever, I don't enjoy the way it makes me feel afterward, as if a part of me is still hiding from feelings I'd be better off to face, as well as wasting my precious dwindling years on a selfish trifle. I've got three kids of my own and a tired wife who needs more help around the house, and a world in need of activism not voyeurism.

All this makes for good PR, of course. But the main reason, I think, has to do with my ma.

Seven years ago, on a sunny day in July, while vacationing with the family in Lake Tahoe, my mother was hit by a truck.

This happened while she was walking to the grocery store to buy ketchup for one or another of her picky grandchildren. The driver didn't see her. His pickup knocked her to the ground.

Her injuries seemed minor initially. She wanted to get right up and keep walking which, fortunately, she was not allowed to do. She wound up in the hospital with internal bleeding and a hairline fracture of her pelvic bone, among other injuries. I mention this because it was really the first time I had seen my mother profoundly incapacitated, her nimble mind blurred by anesthesia.

The following summer, she was diagnosed with cancer, for which she received chemotherapy and underwent the first of two major surgeries. She complained of "chemo brain." But like a lot of intelligent, ambitious people, she managed to conceal the more distressing symptoms. She continued to work as a psychoanalyst. She exercised. She traveled. She published a highly praised book on maternal ambivalence. And we, her loved ones, did our best to attribute her lapses to the general wear and tear one might expect to see in a seventy-five-year-old survivor of multiple cancers.

Then, two summers ago, she began to show more pronounced signs of cognitive decline. In July, she fell on her way to her office to see a patient, and tumbled into a state of delirium. She wound up at an intensive care unit at Stanford Hospital. My wife had just given birth to our third child, but my brothers worried that Mom might be dying and my father admitted he could use some help.

By the time I arrived, my mother's condition had deteriorated. She swung between benign confusion and extreme disorientation. Often, she had no idea where she was and virtually no short-term memory. At one point, she asked where her mother had gone. She insisted she was in the midst of an awful dream and stared in bewilderment at the IVs taped to her arms. Her face was deeply bruised from the fall. She could not feed herself. When doctors asked her basic questions ("Do you know what year it is, Dr. Almond?") she looked at them imploringly.

A nice young doctor sat my dad and me on a bench and told us that the official diagnosis—by which he really meant his best guess—was a progressive dementia that had been masked for years. In the space of a week, she had gone from a high-functioning professional to an invalid who needed around-the-clock monitoring.

One night, as I tried to explain to her for perhaps the tenth time that she could not go home yet, she looked at me in a panic. "Something terrible is happening to me," she said, and began to weep inconsolably.

It was a moment of appalling lucidity. She could see, if only for a few drowning seconds, the true nature of her circumstance.

The next morning, I brought her a picture of her grandson Judah. I thought it might jog her memory, or at least cheer her up. She looked at the photo and began sobbing again.

"What's the matter?" I said.

"I'm going to miss everyone," she said.

The doctors talk about the brain as a mystery. What I realized in those sorrowful days is how holy the brain is. It is a temple that houses our fragile selfhood. We think, therefore we are. But if we cannot think, no matter how vigorous the body, we vanish.

As it turned out, my mom's brain had fooled the docs. Her episode was an acute dementia, apparently triggered in part by medication. Once home, she made a dramatic recovery. She still struggles a bit with short-term memory, and has opted to cut back on her work schedule. Other than that, she's more or less her old self. What we saw was, in effect, a sneak preview of a horror film we're all hoping will never come back to town.

But no one can come face-to-face with dementia and look at football in the same way. At least, I couldn't.

One thing that never ceases to amaze me about America is how much we trumpet our freedom of speech and, at the same time, how little use we make of it, how obedient we are to public consensus. As a population, we generally agree to regard that which is popular as worthy and that which is convenient as necessary. And we shy from even the most obvious statements of truth if they puncture our prevailing myths. Statements such as, *America's economic system incentivizes greed.* Or, *Smart phones are making people stupider.* Or, *It is immoral to watch a sport that causes brain damage.*

Can you recall a single public figure who has ever

condemned football? A major politician? A religious leader? A celebrity of any kind? The most prominent ones are probably Buzz Bissinger and Malcolm Gladwell. Back in 2012, the two of them teamed up to debate the merits of college football against two former players. At the outset of the debate, 16 percent of the audience was in favor of banning the sport in college. Afterward, that figure stood at 53 percent. Gladwell also had the guts to deliver a speech at the University of Pennsylvania a couple of years ago calling for students to boycott football at their school, though he was careful to note that he has no objection to those paid to play professionally.

There is, of course, an entire industry whose ostensible job is to report and comment on the world of sports. But with a few exceptions—most notably, PBS's *Frontline* series and the investigative reporters Mark Fainaru-Wada and Steve Fainaru—the world of sports "journalism" serves as a promotional division of the Athletic Industrial Complex.

If, like me, you are a fan of sports talk radio, you can tune in at any time of the day or night and hear an articulate and passionate discussion of the scandal du jour. Or you can just turn on your TV. The most popular radio shows are now (somewhat amazingly, considering the visuals) televised. In fact, sports punditry is the industry's unrivaled growth sector, a universe of cheaply produced bombast that mimics the dominant form over on the cable "news" networks. Hosts earn their salaries going after almost any form of hypocrisy that might excite their audience: selfish players, incompetent coaches, meddlesome owners.

What sports pundits almost never do is speak about the inherent morality of watching sports, in particular football. They never ask us fans to consider our own complicity in the weekly parade of outrages. Because we fans, by definition at this point, are the victims. We're the ones forever betrayed, ripped off, taken for granted.

One of my favorite sports pundits is Bill Simmons. In fact, he's so good at what he does that it feels unfair to call him a pundit. He captures the joy and agony of fandom in self-effacing prose. He studies our games and offers generous insights. Simmons gets that sports are absurd and, at the same time, deeply meaningful. In the past few years, he's become a TV star and launched a website, Grantland.com, dedicated to the idea that it's possible to write intelligently about sports without being pretentious.

A couple of years ago, Simmons wrote a fascinating column about the bounty scandal mentioned above, in which the defensive coordinator of the New Orleans Saints, Gregg Williams, was caught offering players money for injuring opponents. Here's how that piece concludes:

> *That's what the NFL is banking on these next few years—hypocrisy, basically—as more stories emerge about the tortured lives of retired players. Many of them can't walk, sit down or remember anything. Some battle debilitating headaches and gulp down pills like they're peanuts. A few*

weeks ago, Jim McMahon confessed in an interview that his short-term memory was gone, then admitted he wouldn't even remember the interview as he was giving it. You hear these things, you sigh, you feel remorse, you forget . . . and then you go back to looking forward to the next football season. Gregg Williams crossed the line; he won't be there. I just wish someone would decide, once and for all, where that line really is.

Listen: Bill Simmons is a smart, compassionate guy. And like a lot of smart, compassionate guys, he is genuinely troubled by the damage done to football players. But what he's doing here is pretty bush league. He's performing that old American jujitsu: using acknowledgement of a problem as a form of absolution. He's letting himself, and the rest of us, off the hook.

But Bill Simmons knows the truth: *we* set the line. We, the fans. Not Roger Goodell. Not Congress. Not some squad of avenging lawyers. Us.

And specifically, Bill Simmons. He is, after all, the most influential booster in America, a guy with millions of followers and enough platforms to construct his own sports-themed pagoda. He has more power over the viewing and interpretive habits of fans than any other person in America.

If Bill Simmons declared tomorrow that *he* was drawing the line, that *he* refused to be a hypocrite, that *he* could no longer choose his own viewing pleasure over his conscience, there would be a collective freak-out in the world of American sports. Plenty of fans and players and colleagues would repudiate him. But a lot of others would do some necessary soul-searching. The discussion around football would become—at least in some precincts—a genuine ethical debate rather than an ablution performed before the next big game. At the very least, fans would at last be talking about their true role in the process: as sponsors of the game.

It's not like there's no historical precedent. In 1984, Howard Cosell, the most famous sportscaster in America, called a championship fight between Larry Holmes and Tex Cobb. He was so distressed at the beating Cobb took that he announced, in disgust, that he would never call another fight. He never did. Cosell may have been a raging egotist and a shameless grandstander, but he was also a rarity in the blinkered guild of sportscasters: a man not afraid to draw his own line. Did Cosell's boycott end boxing as we know it? No. That's not the point. You take a stand because it's the right thing to do, not because it's effective.

I don't mean to single out Bill Simmons. There are half a dozen sports pundits smart and principled enough to recognize that football is rotten on all sorts of levels. But when the mics click on, these guys all retreat into a familiar brand of sophistry.

As often as I can, I listen to the opening rant of a guy named Colin Cowherd, who has a national show on ESPN. Cowherd is a terrific orator. He cuts right through the noise of the Athletic Industrial Complex. The guy has a keen bullshit detector. Like a lot of other top-tier hosts, Cowherd dutifully interviewed Mark Fainaru-Wada and Steve Fainaru about their chilling book, *League of Denial*, which details the NFL's repugnant response to the concussion crisis.

But his subsequent rant on the subject of NFL health risks sounded more like an apologia for the league. The real problem, he suggested, was media hype. He made the lives of former players sound like a wonderland of golf tournaments and free buffets. He ran an audio clip of Roger Goodell bragging about how NFL players enjoy longer-than-average lives, never bothering to inform his listeners that this claim is, at best, disputed. Then he ticked through a litany of more dangerous jobs, conveniently neglecting that football players, unlike crane operators, get injured playing a game for the entertainment of fans like him.

The same thing happens every time a new report forces these guys to confront football's dark side. They trot out the same bromides and subtract themselves (and us) from the equation. ESPN's Scott Van Pelt reacted to a *Frontline* documentary on NFL concussions by reminding listeners that players choose this life, and most would do so again. He urged listeners to watch the show with an open mind, then shared his takeaway: "I found myself asking this last night: In what way does what I heard impact me? And the answer, honestly, is it doesn't."

That settles that.

I understand that sports pundits live in the bubble of fandom. It's not just a matter of personal preference. They, and the networks that employ them, are professionally beholden to the NFL. But their rationalizations often devolve into a kind of might-makes-right gospel that feels creepy and frankly fascistic to me. "Football is the most popular thing in America," Scott Van Pelt intoned. "Not the most popular sport. The most popular *thing*."

Van Pelt appeared to believe he was making an ethical argument here, in the same way an oil magnate points to public opinion polls to rebut the science of climate change. To justify belief and behavior based on mass appeal, in the absence of moral consideration, is not democracy. It's mob rule.

Back in 2009, on the Friday before Super Bowl XLIII, Roger Goodell delivered his standard rap about the NFL's commitment to safety before hundreds of media members in a gilded ballroom. An hour later, in a much smaller room just around the corner, a team of independent researchers held a press conference about the realities of CTE. Seven reporters showed up.

This incongruence neatly encapsulates the homerism inherent in sports journalism. But it also raises another question: What about the good old "lame stream" media? How often do they dig beneath the glossy veneer of Big Football?

Not often. This is partly a function of larger trends. Investigative journalism, which is expensive and involves complex subtleties, is in decline. Sports represent one of the few growth sectors for the corporate media. It's far more profitable to cover football as a glorious diversion than a sobering news story.

The executives who run the NFL and NCAA know this. They have the clout to freeze out any reporter, or news organization, that asks inconvenient questions. Like all skilled politicians, Roger Goodell avoids antagonistic media. He has an entire network to disseminate his talking points, after all.

When he does grant access to an outsider, it's always a comfy collaboration. Witness his encounter with Chris Wallace of *Fox News Sunday* before the last Super Bowl. I hesitate to characterize the event as an interview, which would imply critical thought. Wallace came off more like a blushing groupie. His central concern was the weather for the big game. He then moved on to economics, citing Goodell's $25 billion revenue goal. "How do you make the NFL, which seems huge, even bigger?" he gushed. Goodell talked about making football a year-round business and expanding into international markets.

Wallace then asked how Goodell balanced two conflicting priorities, "player safety, *which I guess is foremost*" [emphasis mine] with fans' hunger for big hits. With eleven minutes gone in the twelve-minute spot, Wallace got around to broaching, ever so gently, the issue of brain injuries.

There's no need to print Goodell's answer, which was his usual potion of euphemism, elision, and half-truths. More revealing was the way the session ended, with Wallace asking Goodell to autograph a football "as a keepsake for the Wallace grandchildren."

• • •

Among cultural observers, Chuck Klosterman occupies a fascinating niche. He's an unabashed fan of sports and most other forms of popular culture. He writes excellent literary fiction too. He's a provocative, even contrarian, voice, in part because he appears to be genuinely concerned with ethics.

Here's what he had to say about football after the bounty scandal:

> *Now, I realize an argument can be made that eroticized violence is inherent to any collision spectator sport, and that people who love football are tacitly endorsing (and unconsciously embracing) a barbaric activity that damages human bodies for entertainment and money. I get that, and I don't think the argument is weak.*

Huh?

Why does Chuck Klosterman suddenly sound like a lawyer? Worse, why does he sound like a bureaucrat? This is the nervous prose of someone who wants credit for making a bold moral statement without wanting to feel bound to abide by it. *I get that, and I don't think the argument is weak.*

I've talked to dozens of fans who offer some version of the same concession. Okay, okay, the game is totally corrupt. Can we move on?

In a 2012 column, Klosterman put it like this:

> *Imagine two vertical, parallel lines accelerating skyward—that's what football is like now. On the one hand, there is no*

*way that a cognizant world can continue adoring a game
where the end result is dementia and death; on the other
hand, there is no way you can feasibly eliminate a sport
that generates so much revenue (for so many people) and is
so deeply beloved by everyday citizens who will never have
to absorb the punishment.*

Klosterman writes here with characteristic eloquence.
But there's a logical fallacy deftly tucked away in that last
clause: *there is no way you can feasibly eliminate a sport . . .*

Why the hell not?

Football is a form of entertainment, not a chip that gets
implanted in our necks at birth by the Overlords. Klosterman
is posing as a realist here, but he's being a cynic. He's arguing
that profit and popularity amount to fate in our democracy.

Listen: Moral progress is inconvenient. It destabilizes the
status quo. But the essential task of the American experiment
is to build a more perfect union. Not a more exciting union.
Not an easier, go-with-the-flow union. More perfect. That's
why our citizens fought to end slavery and child labor and
to establish universal suffrage and civil rights and the right
of workers to unionize. Hundreds of thousands died for
these causes.

Are we really so spoiled as a nation, in 2014, that we can't
curb our appetite for an unnecessarily violent game that degrades our educational system, injures its practitioners, and
fattens a pack of gluttonous corporations?

The real problem here (again, tucked away in Klosterman's formulation) is that our citizens refuse to become *cognizant*.

In May, President Obama hosted a summit to raise awareness of concussions in youth sport. It was a quintessentially political gesture: a laudable and largely ceremonial event intended to validate his ardor for the game, which he detailed in a 2013 interview:

I'm a big football fan, but I have to tell you if I had a son, I'd have to think long and hard before I let him play football. And I think that those of us who love the sport are going to have to wrestle with the fact that it will probably change gradually to try to reduce some of the violence. In some cases, that may make it a little bit less exciting, but it will be a whole lot better for the players, and those of us who are fans maybe won't have to examine our consciences quite as much.

A few months later, he added:

I would not let my son play pro football. At this point, there's a little bit of a caveat emptor. These guys, they know what they're doing. They know what they're buying into. It is no longer a secret. It's sort of the feeling I have about smokers, you know?

I don't really know where to begin here. Is the life of Obama's hypothetical son worth more than the lives of the kids who grow into pros? Are players really like smokers? (Do we pack stadiums to watch pro smokers inhale?) Should the final goal of safety reform be to alleviate fan guilt?

Obama may be the one figure in American civic life with the moral authority to put football into its proper perspective. The guy was a community organizer, for God's sake. He battles every day against a roster of billionaires ravenous for corporate welfare, and a public more interested in football scores than his policy goals. And he's not even running for office again.

Couldn't the idealist we elected way back in 2008 awaken from his technocratic trance long enough to draw the line? Would it really be a radical departure from his stated values for him to announce that he can no longer endorse a game that profits by cruelty, that instills avarice, and that harms more than healing our most vulnerable communities? Couldn't the guy at least admit that it's wrong to watch a sport so dangerous he wouldn't let his own son play it?

It is possible that football will grow less popular in this country. After all, boxing was once our top sport. Here's how it might happen:

First, several retired stars might reveal the depth of their neurological impairment. Steve Young on *60 Minutes*. Brett Favre weeping to Oprah. Second, the safer equipment and rules that fans are forever touting as silver bullets may do little to alter the brutal physics of the game. Third, medical technology inevitably will make visible the damage done to young men who play the sport. Fourth, a major college or pro player might be paralyzed or killed during a game. Fifth, a successful class-action suit at the high school or college level could trigger a domino effect.

But realistically, it's going to take more than this to change our collective perception of the game. Cognizance is partly the result of cultural leaders (such as Obama and Simmons and Favre) speaking out, thus refusing to provide us the safe cover of an immoral orthodoxy.

Maybe the way to think of football is as a kind of refuge. Maybe it's so popular because it's the one huge cultural space where we can safely indulge all the shit we haven't worked out yet as a people: our lust for violence, our racial neuroses, our yearning for patriarchal dominion, our sexual hang-ups. It's the place where men get to be boys—before the age of reason, before the age of guilt.

But I keep thinking, also, about this young woman I met the other night, who found out I was writing a book about football and got very excited and told me she was a huge fan of the Philadelphia Eagles, that she had an Eagles hat in her bag, did I want to see it? She told me football was what kept her connected to her hometown, and to her dad especially. "Every weekend he'd go hunting for deer and he'd kill one and make venison burgers and we'd watch the Eagles game. That was our thing."

Her face was shining with love.

"What's your book about, anyway?" she said.

So I did that thing where I marched out all my arguments, which were supposed to make me feel righteous. But I looked at this young woman, at her sad eyes, and all I felt was petty and cruel. The Philadelphia Eagles had given her something precious to share with her father. What right did I have to shit on that?

So I want to say to her, and to you: I'm sorry.

The point of this book isn't to shit on your happiness. It isn't to win some cultural argument. Let's make it larger than that. Let's make it an honest conversation between ourselves, and within ourselves, about why we come to football, about why we need a beautiful savage game to feel fully alive, to feel united, and to love the people we love.

EPILOGUE

STOP BEING A FAN,
START BEING A PLAYER

How much easier it is to be critical than to be correct.

—Benjamin Disraeli

Readers may come away from this book with the reasonable objection that it's long on questions and complaints and short on solutions. It was so designed. My intention was to inveigle readers—fans and non-fans alike—into a state of distress and contemplation. Best to understand the illness before we seek the cure.

That being said, there are practical steps that can and should be taken to address the most glaring moral hazards football presents. The following list represents not a blueprint so much as an effort to instigate discussion. If you agree with any of these measures, make your voice heard by those with the power to propose and legislate.

• *Revoke the NFL's non-profit status*

Should have been done forty years ago.

• *Require that allocation of public funds for sports facilities
be approved by public referendum*

In 1997, Pittsburghers voted down a referendum that
would have imposed a sales tax to build the Steelers a new
stadium. Despite public uproar, the city came up with a "Plan
B"—widely known as *Scam B*—by which the taxpayers ponied
up more than $200 million while team ownership chipped in
$76 million. The Heinz Company promptly paid *the owners*
$57 million for naming rights.

The will of the voters should never be subverted by back-
room deals.

Likewise, city and county officials should pass measures
that require sports franchises to share the profits derived from
the facilities where they play, based on the percentage of public funding.

• *Institute a parental discretion warning before football games*

Films are rated based, in part, on acts of simulated violence. Football games contain hundreds of acts of real violence, the most extreme replayed ad nauseam. Why not force
parents to confront this upfront?

• *Enforce a weight limit on players and/or teams*

A study published in the *Journal of the American Medical Association* reported that 56 percent of all pro players who suited up during the 2003 season had a body mass index doctors would consider overweight. Players gorge themselves to put on pounds, especially in light of the NFL's crackdown on steroids. Retired lineman Brad Culpepper explains: "Now you have to be 300 to move people." Players at every position have gotten bigger, making collisions more damaging, and increasing the risks of heart disease, stroke, diabetes, etc.

A weight limit at the pro level—either for individual positions, or for a team *in toto*—would compel players to slim down rather than bulk up, an incentive that would slim down the college and high school game as well.

• *Create a helmet that records every sub-concussive hit*

Most medical experts agree that there is no way around the basic physics of football: players colliding at high speeds cause brain traumas. No magic helmet is going to change that.

However, as researchers at the University of North Carolina and Purdue have shown, the technology does exist to measure the overall impact absorbed by a particular player. So why not monitor impact and mandate benching players who amass too many Gs? This would create an incentive for coaches and players to avoid the style of play ("Lead with your head, son!") that results in brain injuries.

- *Include graduation rates in a college team's national ranking*

My own "solution" to college football would be to eliminate it in favor of a non-profit developmental league—overseen by a public trust—for players from eighteen to twenty-two years old.

But the above suggestion, one of several derived from Gregg Easterbrook's excellent book *The King of Sports*, would at least begin to reform the college game, by forcing coaches to make sure players (most of whom will not go pro) earn a diploma. Easterbrook also recommends that the NCAA suspend any head coach for one year if his team graduation rate dips below that of the general student population at his school.

- *Prohibit tackle football for high schoolers younger than sixteen*

My hope is that lawsuits will eventually induce high schools to drop football altogether. Until then, at least make students wait a couple of years before they play Russian roulette with their brain function. Junior varsity squads can play flag football. Practice time, for all students, should be limited. And no spring football.

- *Require a 3.0 GPA to play varsity football*

As at the college level, this is the only way to make sure players (and coaches) get serious about academics, and would have the added benefit of influencing coaches at the youth level.

Would this be hard on some players? Yes. But ignoring their intellectual development is a far greater injustice.

• *Remember who's in charge*

It's easy to forget this, but fans are the ones who have given football the awesome power it holds. We can, and should, use that power to reshape the game in ways that make it less destructive to the bodies of the players, to the economic fate of our cities, and to the national soul.

If you agree that the time has come to reclaim this power, please help keep the conversation going. Offer a suggestion of your own, or an anecdote, or simply make your voice heard at www.againstfootball.org.

SUDDEN DEATH: AN ODD BUT NECESSARY AFTERWORD

Football Is Dead! Long Live Football!

One morning in the fall of 2014, just days after the initial publication of this book, I burst into the kitchen, where my wife, Erin, was finishing up a bagel abandoned by one of our many children and quietly hoping I would not bring up football. I had for weeks been bursting into various rooms in our home to inflict upon her news of the scandals suddenly engulfing the National Football League.

"Honey, you're never going to believe what *The New York Times* just reported!" I announced.

"Is it about the guy who hit his girlfriend?"

She meant Ray Rice, the Baltimore Ravens running back who had been captured on a surveillance camera knocking his fiancée unconscious.

"No."

"Is it about the guy who beat his son?"

She meant Adrian Peterson, an even more famous

running back who had been arrested for whipping his three-year-old with a thin branch.

"No," I said. "This is bigger. Much bigger."

Erin looked at me. *Though I am very tired and do not actually care*, this look said, *I will let you tell me because you are my husband and I have no choice.* It is from this humble fabric of patience that marriages are made.

The breaking news? Actuarial experts hired by the NFL had just estimated that 30 percent of its retired players would suffer "long-term cognitive ailments." This figure was especially shocking because league officials had spent decades denying any link between football and brain injuries. "I don't see how football survives this," I told my wife. "You can't have a third of the employees in America's most famous workplace suffering brain damage. That's just not a sustainable model. Americans won't stand for it."

I respectfully request that you stop laughing.

A few days later, I found myself seated in a refrigerated cable news studio in the middle of Manhattan, preparing (I assumed) to discuss the NFL's stunning revelation. Alas, my lavishly caffeinated host had a different hook in mind. She was concerned about when Adrian Peterson might be allowed to play football again.

•   •   •

Still, "FOOTBALL IN CRISIS" was the banner headline of the sports world during the 2014 season. *Time* magazine put a picture of a high school player on its cover, moments before he was killed on the field, accompanied by the headline, "IS FOOTBALL WORTH IT?" If you were the sort of heartbroken idiot who buys into such things, you might actually have believed, at least for a few weeks, that America was ready to confront the profound corruptions of its Football Industrial Complex.

But the raging inferno turned out to be little more than a campfire into which fans peered for a few unsettling segments before returning to the true business of fandom, which is to escape from the complexities of adulthood into passionate and childish tribalism. The ratings for the NFL and college football were higher than ever last season. En route to its own funeral, football had been resurrected.

It worked like this:

First, the folks with the microphones focused obsessively on individual moral actors. Nearly all the coverage concerned Rice and Peterson and whether the league was doing enough to punish them. In this way, the narrative of "NFL violence" was safely channeled into designated scapegoats, whose outbursts occurred off the field.

The nature of the crimes was so disturbing—and the visual evidence of them so alluring—that fans were encouraged to see themselves as victims by proxy, not just of Rice and of Peterson, but of NFL commissioner Roger Goodell. The idea seemed to be that Goodell's expulsion would cleanse the league of its sins, as opposed to ushering in some new corporate impresario to stage-manage them.

Nobody asked the obvious question: to what extent did the violent and impulsive culture of football contribute to these violent, impulsive crimes?

I kept trying to imagine what would happen if some other major employer—McDonald's, for instance, or Microsoft, or the U.S. Army—announced that nearly a third of its employees were likely to develop brain damage. How big would the ensuing political-media-consumer freak-out be?

This was part of my effort to understand how football had become exempt from our collective standards of decency. But the analogy made no sense. Because the relationship we have with football players is so intimate. We don't think of them as employees, but as gods. We worship them for the miracles their bodies create. They inhabit us spiritually. To view the gridiron strictly as a workplace is to ignore its religious functions.

And yet, once we enter the realm of faith, rational thought and moral imagination are the first casualties. We find ourselves cleaving to myth and magic, so as to ward off the disruptive notion that our heroic amusement might represent the darker impulses of the national soul. Or worse, the perversion of our own.

The radio host Colin Cowherd provided a chilling example in his response to the Ray Rice affair. He blamed the savagery of our popular culture—video games, songs, movies. These, he insisted, "lead to aggression, desensitization toward violence, a lack of sympathy for victims, and particularly in kids."

Conspicuously absent from his list was football. Here, then, was the myth. The magic resided in the notion that our most popular and profitable sport was actually the only thing keeping the lower castes from revolt. For supporting evidence, Cowherd played an audio clip of Hall of Fame linebacker Ray Lewis. Lewis was asked what would happen if NFL players went on strike. "Watch how much evil, which we call crime, picks up if you take away our game," he warned.

"I don't know if he's right or not," Cowherd said.

It is worth pausing here a long moment to ponder what it means that a national radio host would stoop to this kind of fearmongering. And that he would offer such menacing testimony from a man who, in addition to working as an ESPN analyst, was almost charged with murder for his role in a street brawl that took place a few hours after the 2000 Super Bowl.

Such tortured logic epitomized the prevailing discourse. Everywhere you turned, pundits were howling about football.

And yet the essential aim of these lamentations was to preserve the status quo, in which Americans could consume a lethal game without suffering the burden of complicity and guilt.

A week into the new season, the British newspaper *The Guardian* published a column click-baitishly headlined, "DOES WATCHING THE NFL MAKE YOU EVIL?" and accompanied online by a link that read: "NFL week one preview—with Pick Six contest."

The column's author, Jeb Lund, was more refined in his rhetoric than Cowherd, and more robust in his indignation. "Given its indifference toward women and racism, its eagerness to plunder public coffers and its outright economic and medical hostility toward its own labor force, it is flabbergasting that any of us remain fans of the NFL at all," Lund wrote. "It's a game of on-the-field supermen managed and exploited with all the 'superman' sociopathy of Wall Street–Silicon Valley vulture capital neofascism." Lund was *really* disgusted with the NFL. So disgusted that his very next paragraph read as follows: "I will probably watch over 300 hours of this game before the postseason starts."

Which brings me to the most common question I received as the author of a book titled *Against Football*:

"Wait, you mean you're actually going to *stop* watching football?"

•   •   •

There were other reactions, of course. One kindly troll suggested that I be turned over to ISIS for beheading. A woman writing for the *Los Angeles Times* suggested that my problem wasn't with football but "with maleness itself."

As for the critics, the approach taken by *Esquire*'s Tom Junod was representative. "I know but one thing about the upcoming football season," he wrote. "I'm going to watch it. And I'm going to feel a little bad about watching it." His goal wasn't to engage the arguments set forth in this book, but to inoculate himself from them.

Another reviewer reassured readers that "football seems to be able to adjust to new concerns as they arise." He cited the NFL's hefty donation to a brain research center as proof of its compassion for players, ignoring the fact that 5,000 of them had joined a suit accusing the NFL of negligence and fraud. The piece functioned as a press release from league headquarters. It was published by *The Washington Post*.

At times, I found myself thinking about it from the point of view of the brains. The brain inside Janay Palmer was rendered insensate by her partner Ray Rice. Millions of Americans watched replays of this neurological event and reacted with horror and outrage. Every weekend, the brains inside numerous NFL players were rendered insensate by fellow players. Millions of Americans watched replays of these neurological events, as well, and reacted with fascination and sometimes glee.

What's the logical conclusion here, if you're a brain?

It must be that Americans feel some persistent and largely unexamined emotional need to watch you suffer traumatic injury.

The other major media narrative last season, you'll recall, involved the deaths of two unarmed African-American men, Eric Garner and Michael Brown, at the hands of white police officers, none of whom were indicted.

Darren Wilson, the officer who fired six bullets into Brown, told the grand jury that during an initial tussle he "felt like a five-year-old holding on to to Hulk Hogan." He feared Brown could have killed him with a punch to the face. "The only way I can describe it," Wilson noted of Brown's expression, "it looked like a demon, that's how angry he looked." Brown stood six feet, four inches, and weighed 290 pounds. Wilson (the five-year-old) was the same height and weighed 210 pounds.

White Americans, of course, have a long history of demonizing African-American men as physically monstrous to justify violence against them as defensive in nature. And yet it was difficult to read Wilson's testimony and not wonder to what extent our addiction to football reinforces these grotesque stereotypes. Isn't the essential racial paradox of football that mostly white fans cheer players who are mostly African-American, young men whose superhuman strength and preternatural aggression we secretly view as inbred rather than cultivated by our regard?

The Garner arrest was even more distressing. Video of the incident showed Officer Daniel Pantaleo attempting to cuff Garner for the grand crime of selling loose cigarettes. When Garner pushed his hands away, Pantaleo jumped on his back and applied a fatal chokehold. Three other officers helped gang-tackle Garner—six-three and 350 pounds—to the ground. Garner gasped "I can't breathe" eleven times. He was dead within minutes.

The footage looks like a gridiron sequence as choreographed by Jim Crow, right down to Pantaleo's wardrobe.

He isn't wearing police blues. He's wearing a football jersey.

I suspect I'll catch hell for drawing this connection. But I'm tired of pretending that our avid and endless consumption of football doesn't shape how we see the world. We know what football does for us. The scarier and more important question is what does it do *to* us.

A few other updates are in order.

As predicted, my Oakland Raiders went 3–13 in 2014. That earned them the fourth pick in the draft, which means they missed out on Heisman Trophy winner and accused rapist

Jameis Winston, who went number one overall. Richie In-cognito, last seen harassing his teammate Jonathan Martin, signed on with the Buffalo Bills. Adrian Peterson will be back in uniform, too. That's the law in the jungle of capitalism. Workers of sufficient talent will always find a willing bidder.

Unless, of course, you get yourself arrested for murder, which happened to Aaron Hernandez, the New England Pa-triots' star tight end. I was on a JetBlue flight when the verdict was announced, and virtually every TV onboard was tuned to the coverage, an endless tape loop of Hernandez skulking off in shackles.

I returned to the book I was reading, the George Plimp-ton classic *Mad Ducks and Bears*. I had reached the part where an offensive lineman named John Gordy explains to the au-thor why he returned to pro football after being driven from the game by nervous anxiety:

> "Oh Christ!" he said. "The best thing in football was to really pop someone. One of the great joys of my life was to get a bead on a guy and really put him out. Absolutely! To lift him up right under his chin, or un-der his throat with the top of your helmet and put him on his back on the grass. You've done your job, you've gotten your good grade. The movie's going to show it. That's it. Yes, that's why I came back to the Lions the next year."

Hernandez will spend his remaining years in prison, where, chances are, he will live a longer and healthier life than his teammates who did not commit murder.

There was one other major football story last season, which involved a star linebacker named Chris Borland, who gobsmacked the sports world by quitting at age twenty-four after a remarkable rookie season, citing concerns about brain disease. He feared that unless he left the game, its ruthless code of valor (and corresponding financial incentives) would overrule his common sense.

In the course of making his decision, Borland consulted with Dave Meggyesy, a linebacker who quit the NFL in 1969, arguing that football conditioned Americans to tolerate violence and racism in other contexts, particularly the Vietnam War. Meggyesy's 1971 memoir, *Out of Their League*, portrayed the game, from the inside, as a kind of factory designed to mold young men into weapons.

This critique was far more radical than the statements Borland made. But both men were, in their own ways, rebelling against football's deepest form of indoctrination, which is the idea that courage resides in a man's willingness to visit harm upon another man, and to quietly absorb it.

What about refusing to participate in a sport that slowly maims you, or that diminishes your humanity? Isn't that a form of courage as well?

• • •

Borland was careful to emphasize that he wasn't telling anyone else what to do. He just wanted kids and parents to make "an informed decision" about whether to play football.

The whole point of *Against Football* is to help *fans* make an informed decision about football. In the course of composing the book, I was forced to connect a lot of the dots that had remained happily unconnected for years. Having done so, I decided to turn away from football, a game I still adore.

But that's just me. What matters here is you. There is no "right" response to this book. There is only your response.

Just this morning, *The New York Times* published a story about Patrick Risha, a college football player whose psychological and cognitive struggles led him to commit suicide at the age of thirty-two, while on the phone with his mother. Risha's brain showed degenerative illness of the sort commonly found in ex-players. The piece, titled "A Son of Football Calls His Mother," ran on the front page of the Sports section. It was, in fact, the only story on the page, hovering in a sea of ghostly white.

This marks the first time a major newspaper has ever presented such an account in a manner undiluted by the usual deluge of promotional copy (draft previews, free agent signings, etc.). The editors at the *Times* were saying, in effect, this: We refuse to treat football solely as a form of entertainment; it is also a moral undertaking with real human consequences.

The story is painful to read, and therefore inconvenient. It is also a small but vital sign of progress.

When society changes in the way I hope it will, football will be obsolete.

That's what Dave Meggyesy said nearly fifty years ago.

It's more or less how I feel today.

I recognize this marks me as a dreamer and a fool. And a hypocrite and a loudmouth. What can I tell you? I believe in nonviolent action and social justice, all that crap Christ spouted on the Mount. I see the riots raging in American cities as the sad but inevitable result of a system rigged against poor kids, many of them African-American. I don't see football as a cure for these ills. I see it as part of a larger mind-set that regards certain lives as disposable, unless they are housed in bodies that happen to be able to entertain us.

Football isn't our destiny. It's not some spectacle we have to stage to keep the seething masses opiated. It's just a game, one we use to find grace and meaning and common ground with other fans.

Those are all lovely human pursuits. But they can be achieved by other means, ones that don't force us to crouch behind delusion as we sponsor cruelty, as we squander the human virtue most worth defending, which is mercy.